THE CHICKEN HEALTH BIBLE

The Most Comprehensive Guide to Ensuring Your Flock Health and Defeating Diseases in Chickens of All Breeds and Ages

Noah Phipps

Copyright © 2023 Noah Phipps

All rights reserved.

No part of this publication may be reproduced, stored in a retrieval system, stored in a database, and / or published in any form or by any means, electronic, mechanical, photocopying, recording, or otherwise, without the prior written permission of the publisher.

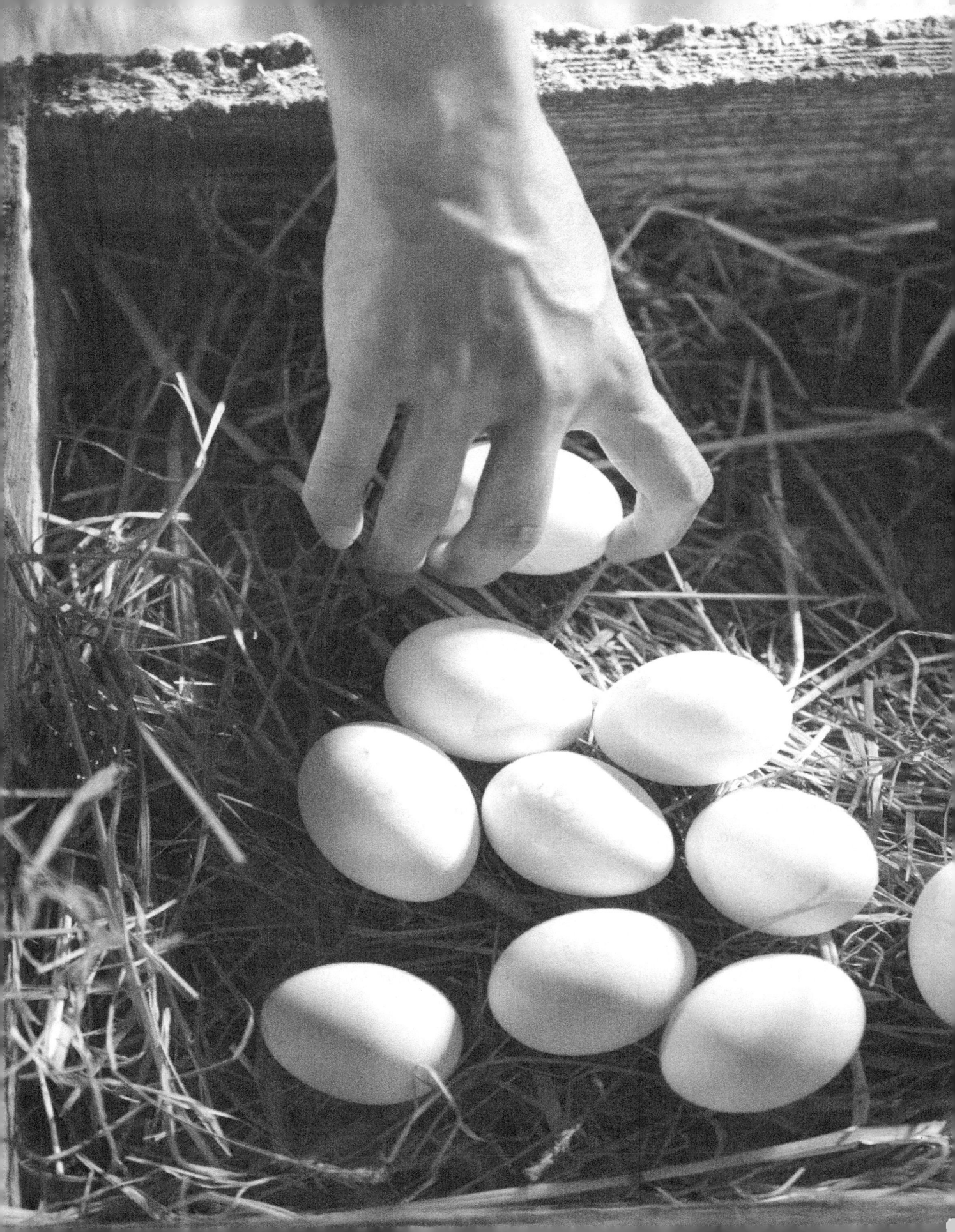

The Chicken Health Bible

"With decades of experience and a deep passion for poultry, Phipps has masterfully crafted a guide that stands in a league of its own. His profound knowledge shines through every page, delivering invaluable insights and practical advice that transcend conventional poultry care."

- **Backyard Poultry Magazine**

"Within the pages of this exceptional guide lies a wealth of knowledge that poultry enthusiasts and chicken lovers alike simply cannot ignore. The Chicken Health Bible is a masterpiece, written with impeccable precision and attention to detail."

- **Farming Magazine**

"This opus stands tall as the definitive guide to maintaining the health and conquering diseases in chickens of all breeds and ages."

- **Countryside Magazine**

"From preventative care to conquering diseases, this book's carefully curated content will transform your understanding of chicken health. Impeccably written, it is a testament to the author's expertise and passion for poultry well-being."

- **Sustainable Farming Magazine**

"The book leaves no aspect of poultry health untouched, ensuring you possess the necessary tools to combat diseases and promote the vitality of your cherished flock."

- **Hobby Poultry Magazine**

Table of Contents

INTRODUCTION 13

CHAPTER 1: BACKYARD FLOCK HEALTH AND COMFORTABLE 15
    The Backyard Chicken: 15
    Creating a Healthy Life for Your Flock 15
  CLEANING AND DISINFECTING 101 16
    Cleaning and Disinfecting in Construction: 17
    The Art of Cleaning: 17
    How to Make a Good Disinfection: 17
    Safely Using and Disposing of Disinfectants: 18
    Chicken Health Bible and Cleaning: 18
  PROVIDING A HEALTHY AND COMFORTABLE ENVIRONMENT 19
    Cleaning and Disinfecting the Chicken Coop: 19
    Creating Comfy Bedding: 19
    Handling Outdoor Runs: 20
    Managing Adverse Weather Events: 20
  KEEP YOUR FLOCK FIT 21
    Common Health Problems in Chickens 21
    Major Causes of Death in Chickens 21
    Safely Sourcing New Birds 21

CHAPTER 2: HEALTHY CHICKEN BEHAVIOR 23
  THE CHICKEN DAILY ROUTINE 24
    How to Start the Day: 24
    How to Settle in for the Night: 24
    How to Be Together in the Flock: 25
  HOW TO KEEP PEACE IN THE FLOCK 25
    The Role of the Rooster: 25
    Establishing Hierarchies: 25
    Managing Sibling Rivalry: 26
  HOW CHICKENS COMMUNICATE 27
    The Role of Roosters in Communication: 27
    The Chatter of Hens: 27
    Talking Among Themselves: 27
    Courtship Behaviors: 28

CHAPTER 3: BIOSECURITY FOR THE BACKYARD FLOCK 29

How's Your Biosecurity?	29
Recognizing How Disease Is Spread in Chicken Flocks	29
A Big Risk: The New Chicken (or the New Egg)	29
The Other Risks: People, Other Animals, and Equipment	30
Potential Critters in Chicken Feed	30
Implementing Biosecurity Measures	30
A BIOSECURITY PLAN	31
Importance of Biosecurity:	31
Biosecurity Habits in Daily Chores:	31
Biosecurity for Show Chickens:	31

CHAPTER 4: FOOD SAFETY AND QUALITY OF HOMEGROWN EGGS AND MEAT 33

How to Properly Handle Eggs:	33
Managing Layers and Nests:	34
To Wash or Not to Wash?	34
How to Inspect and Store Eggs:	34
SAFE HIGH-QUALITY MEAT FROM YOUR OWN FLOCK	35
Choosing and Preparing Your Birds:	35
How to Prepare the Work Area:	35
Sanitizing Between Birds:	36
How to Inspect Your Processed Chickens:	36
Passing Judgment:	36
Chillin' the Chicken:	36
How to Prepare and Store the Meat:	36

CHAPTER 5: GOOD NUTRITION FOR HEALTHY CHICKEN 39

YOUR CHICKENS' NUTRITIONAL NEEDS	40
Protein:	40
Carbohydrates:	40
Fats:	40
Vitamins:	40
Minerals:	41
Water:	41
Grit:	41
Treats and Supplements:	41
NUTRITIONAL NEEDS OF DIFFERENT LIFE STAGES	41
Chick Stage:	42
Grower Stage:	42
Layer Stage:	42
Senior Stage:	42
Special Considerations:	42
STARTER FEED/BABY FOOD: 0-8 WEEKS	43
Importance of Proper Nutrition:	43
Choosing the Right Starter Feed:	43
Feeding Schedule and Practices:	44
Starter Feed Introduction:	44
Consulting the Chicken Health Bible:	44

GROWER FEED/PULLET FOOD: 8-16 WEEKS 44
    The Importance of Grower Feed: 44
    Composition of Grower Feed: 45
    Benefits of Grower Feed: 45
    Feeding Recommendations: 45

LAYER FEED FOR HENS: 16 WEEKS AND UP 46
    Understanding Layer Feed: 46
    Composition of Layer Feed: 46
    Benefits of Layer Feed: 46
    Feeding Recommendations: 47

THE IMPORTANCE OF GRIT 47
    Disease Prevention: 47
    Emergency Response: 48
    Problem Solving: 48
    Adaptability: 48
    Emotional Resilience: 48

GRAINS & GOODIES 48

WHAT NOT TO FEED 50
    Processed Foods: 50
    Toxic Plants: 50
    Avocado: 50
    Chocolate and Caffeine: 50
    Onions and Garlic: 50
    Citrus Fruits: 51
    Raw Beans: 51

CARBOHYDRATES 51
    Understanding Carbohydrates: 51
    Functions of Carbohydrates: 51
    Sources of Carbohydrates: 52
    Benefits of Carbohydrates in Chicken Diets: 52

FATS 52
    Energy Source: 53
    Nutrient Absorption: 53
    Essential Fatty Acids: 53
    Feather Quality: 53
    Palatability and Diet Formulation: 53

PROTEINS 54
    Essential for Growth and Development: 54
    Of Bodily Functions: 54
    Source of Energy: 54

VITAMINS & MINERALS 55
    Vitamins: 55
    Minerals: 55

WATER 56
    Hydration and Body Functions: 56
    Nutrient Absorption: 56

    Digestion and Gut Health: 57
    Temperature Regulation: 57
    Immune System Support: 57

CHAPTER 6: ANATOMY AND BODY FUNCTIONS — 59

    Eyes, ears, skin, and feathers 60
    Breathing and circulating blood 61
    Eating and digestion 62
    Digestive System of Chickens: 62
    Promoting Healthy Digestion: 63

THE SKELETAL SYSTEM — 63
    Structure and Composition: 63
    Functions of the Skeletal System: 64
    Common Skeletal Issues in Chickens: 64
    Maintaining Skeletal Health: 64

THE CHICKEN AND THEN THE EGG — 65
    Growth and Development: 65
    Reaching Sexual Maturity: 65
    Making Eggs (and Chicks, maybe): 65
    Knowing what goes on in the egg: 65
    A Chick's First Few Weeks: 65

CHAPTER 7: SIGNS OF CHICKEN ILLNESS — 67

RECOGNIZING THE GENERAL SIGNS OF ILLNESS — 68
    Changes in behavior: 68
    Abnormal droppings: 68
    Respiratory issues: 68
    Changes in appearance: 68
    Changes in egg production: 69

THE PHYSICAL EXAMINATION — 69
    Importance of Physical Examination: 69
    Components of a Physical Examination: 69

CATCHING AND HOLDING THE SICK CHICKEN — 70
    Observe and Assess: 70
    Gather Supplies: 70
    Approach Calmly: 71
    Secure the Chicken: 71
    Provide Support and Comfort: 71
    Minimize Stress: 71
    Seek Veterinary Assistance: 71

EXAMINING THE HEAD — 71
    The Head as a Window to Overall Health: 72
    Key Areas of Examination: 72
    Common Head-Related Health Conditions: 72
    Prevention and Care: 73

LOOKING AT SKIN AND FEATHERS — 73

LOOKING AT WINGS, LEGS, AND FEET — 74

  The Wings: _____ 74
  The Legs: _____ 74
  The Feet: _____ 75
 CHECKING THE ABDOMEN AND VENT _____ 75
  Importance of Abdomen and Vent Examination: _____ 75
  How to Check the Abdomen and Vent: _____ 76

CHAPTER 8: COMMON ILLNESSES IN ADULT CHICKENS _____ 77

  Diagnosing Chicken Respiratory Illness: _____ 77
  Giving Supportive Care for Chicken Respiratory Illness: _____ 78
 DIARRHEA IN ADULT CHICKENS _____ 78
  Diagnosing Diarrhea in Adult Chickens: _____ 78
  Giving Supportive Care for Adult Chickens with Diarrhea: _____ 79
 EGG-BINDING AND VENT PROLAPSE _____ 80
  Identifying Egg-Binding: _____ 80
  Identifying Vent Prolapse: _____ 80
  Treatment and Care: _____ 80
 EGG QUALITY ISSUES _____ 81
  Finding the Cause of Egg Quality Issues: _____ 81
  Handling Odd-Shaped Eggs with Care: _____ 82
 POOR SIGHT AND SORE EYES _____ 82
  Potential Eye Problems in Chickens: _____ 82
  Treatments for Eye Issues in Chickens: _____ 83
 SKIN PROBLEMS AND FEATHER LOSS _____ 83
  Soothing skin problems: _____ 84
 DIZZY CHICKEN AND OTHER ALARMING SIGNS _____ 85
 LEG AND FOOT ISSUES _____ 86
  Bumblefoot: _____ 86
  Leg Mites: _____ 86
  Leg Injuries: _____ 86
  Vitamin and Mineral Deficiencies: _____ 87
  Gout: _____ 87

CHAPTER 9: SICK CHICKS _____ 89

  Spotting Problems of the Newly Hatched: _____ 89
  Finding Reasons for Chick Malformations: _____ 89
  Straightening Spraddle Legs: _____ 90
  Singing the Belly-Button Blues: _____ 90
  Unpasting a Pasty Vent: _____ 90
 PROBLEMS OF GROWING CHICKENS _____ 91
  Respiratory Problems: _____ 91
  Diarrhea in Young Chickens: _____ 91
  Nervous System Illnesses in Young Chickens: _____ 91

CHAPTER 10: CHICKEN PARASITES _____ 93

 INTERNAL PARASITES _____ 94

Coccidiosis:	94
Parasitic Worms:	94
Other Internal Parasites:	95
EXTERNAL PARASITES	96
Poultry Lice:	96
Mites:	96
Chiggers, Fleas, and Bedbugs:	97

CHAPTER 11: DISEASES CAUSED BY PROTOZOA — 99

COCCIDIOSIS:	99
HISTOMONIASIS (BLACKHEAD DISEASE):	99
TRICHOMONIASIS:	100
TOXOPLASMOSIS:	100
GIARDIASIS:	100

CHAPTER 12: DISEASES CAUSED BY BACTERIA AND VIRUSES — 101

DISEASES CAUSED BY BACTERIA	101
Avian Intestinal Spirochetosis:	102
Avian Tuberculosis:	102
Colibacillosis (E. coli Infections):	102
Fowl Cholera:	102
Infectious Coryza:	102
Mycoplasmosis:	103
Necrotic Enteritis:	103
Pullorum Disease and Fowl Typhoid:	103
DISEASES CAUSED BY VIRUSES	103
Avian Encephalomyelitis:	103
Avian Influenza:	103
Chicken Infectious Anemia:	104
Fowl Pox:	104
Infectious Bronchitis:	104
Infectious Bursal Disease:	104
Infectious Laryngotracheitis:	104
Lymphoid Leukosis:	104
Marek's Disease:	105
Newcastle Disease:	105

CHAPTER 13: FUNGUS AND MYSTERY DISEASES FUNGAL INFECTIONS — 107

MOLDS AND YEASTS	108
Brooder Pneumonia (Aspergillosis):	108
Candidiasis (Thrush):	109
Ringworm (Favus):	109
OTHER DISEASES WITH MYSTERIOUS CAUSES	110
Broiler Breakdowns:	110
Bumblefoot (Pododermatitis):	110
Crop Problems:	110
Gout and Kidney Stones:	110

    Misfires of the Reproductive Tract: 111

CHAPTER 14: FLOCK MANAGEMENT AND ACCIDENTS 113

DEFENDING AGAINST PREDATORS 114
- The Air Attack: 114
- The Ground Assault: 114

FLOCK-MATE PERSECUTION OR CANNIBALISM 115
- Causes of Flock-Mate Persecution and Cannibalism: 115
- Prevention and Correction Strategies: 116

NUTRITIONAL DISORDERS 117
- Obesity in Chickens: 117
- Excess Calcium: 117
- Vitamin and Mineral Deficiencies: 117

HOW TO RECOGNIZE SOURCES OF POISONINGS IN YOUR BACKYARD 118
- Botulism: 118
- Household Poisons: 118
- Lead Poisoning: 118
- Mold Toxins in Feed (Mycotoxins): 118
- Toxic Gas: 119
- Toxic Foods and Plants: 119

HOW TO IDENTIFY HOUSING AND ENVIRONMENTAL DANGERS 119
- Frostbite: Hardware Disease: 119
- Heat Stress: 120
- Starve-outs: 120
- Suffocation: 120

CHAPTER 15: DIAGNOSTIC GUIDES 121

GETTING ADVICE OR GOING IT ALONE 122

HOW TO COLLECT SAMPLES FOR YOUR CHICKEN-HEALTH ADVISOR 124

HOW TO PERFORM A DIY POSTMORTEM 125
- Gathering Equipment: 125
- Getting Started: 126
- Necropsy of a Chicken: 126

CHAPTER 16: MEDICATING AND VACCINATING BACKYARD FLOCKS 129
- The Link between Drugs and Food-Producing Animals: 130
- Regulations and Guidelines: 130
- Responsible Antibiotic Use: 130
- Vaccination: 131

TO VACCINATE OR NOT TO VACCINATE? PROS AND CONS 131
- Pros of Vaccinating Backyard Chickens: 132
- Cons of Vaccinating Backyard Chickens: 132
- Vaccinating Successfully: 132

MEDICATIONS AND VACCINATIONS 133
- Medications and Vaccinations in Drinking Water: 133
- Medications and Vaccinations by Mouth: 133

    Medications and Vaccinations via Eyedrop: _____ 134
    Medications and Vaccinations through Wing Web Stab: _____ 134
    Medications and Vaccinations Under the Skin (Subcutaneous Injection): _____ 134
    Medications and Vaccinations in the Muscle (Intramuscular Injection): _____ 135

CHAPTER 17: CHICKEN FIRST AID   137

    Assessing the Situation: _____ 137
    Basic First Aid Supplies: _____ 137
    Common Injuries and Illnesses: _____ 138
    Emergency Care: _____ 138
    Preventive Measures: _____ 138

CHAPTER 18: YOUR CHICKENS AND YOUR HEALTH   141

    Physical Health Benefits: _____ 141
    Emotional and Mental Well-being: _____ 142
    Potential Risks and Precautions: _____ 142

  BACTERIAL INFECTIONS YOU CAN GET FROM CHICKENS _____ 143
    Prevention and Control Measures: _____ 143

  WHAT YOU CAN GET FROM CLEANING CHICKEN COOPS _____ 144

  HOW TO PROTECT YOURSELF _____ 145
    Biosecurity Measures: _____ 145
    Vaccinations: _____ 146
    Nutritional Health: _____ 146
    Parasite Control: _____ 146
    Environmental Considerations: _____ 146
    Early Detection and Treatment: _____ 146
    Education and Networking: _____ 147

CONCLUSION   149

Introduction

Welcome to the Chicken Health Bible, your comprehensive guide to ensuring the well-being and vitality of your feathered friends. Whether you are a seasoned poultry keeper or a beginner venturing into the world of backyard chickens, this resource is designed to provide you with essential knowledge and practical tips to keep your flock in optimum health.

Caring for chickens goes beyond simply providing them with food and shelter. Just like any other living beings, chickens are susceptible to a range of health issues and diseases. Understanding their unique biology, recognizing common ailments, and implementing preventive measures are crucial for maintaining a happy and thriving flock.

In the Chicken Health Bible, we have compiled a wealth of information to empower you as a chicken owner. From basic anatomy and physiology to nutrition and disease prevention, we cover a wide range of topics relevant to chicken health. You will learn about the signs of a healthy chicken, how to create a comfortable coop environment, and the importance of a balanced diet.

Furthermore, this guide delves into the most common health problems that can affect your chickens, including respiratory issues, parasites, bacterial and viral infections, and reproductive disorders. We provide valuable insights into identifying symptoms, implementing appropriate treatments, and taking preventive measures to minimize the risk of these conditions.

To ensure the accuracy and reliability of the information presented, the Chicken Health Bible draws upon the expertise of experienced poultry veterinarians, researchers, and seasoned chicken keepers. Our aim is to empower you with practical knowledge and empower you to make informed decisions when it comes to the health and well-being of your flock.

Remember, healthy chickens are happy chickens, and a thriving flock will reward you with delicious eggs, delightful companionship, and a fulfilling backyard experience. So, let's dive into the pages of the Chicken Health Bible and embark on a journey to nurture the health of your feathered companions like never before.

Chapter 1

Backyard Flock Health And Comfortable

Welcome to the Chicken Health Bible! This comprehensive guide aims to provide you with the knowledge and tools to ensure the health and comfort of your backyard flock. In this first chapter, we will focus on the basics of maintaining a healthy and comfortable environment for your chickens. By implementing these practices, you can promote their overall well-being, prevent diseases, and maximize their productivity.

The Backyard Chicken:

In recent years, backyard chicken keeping has gained tremendous popularity. More and more people are recognizing the benefits of having a small flock of chickens in their own backyard. These charming birds not only provide fresh eggs but also offer companionship and a unique connection to nature. However, to fully enjoy the rewards of backyard chicken keeping, it is crucial to prioritize the health and comfort of your feathered friends.

Creating a Healthy Life for Your Flock

1. **Housing and Space:** Providing a suitable housing environment is essential for the health and comfort of your chickens. A well-designed coop should protect them from predators, harsh weather conditions, and excessive noise. It should be spacious enough to allow each chicken to have at least 4 square feet of indoor space and sufficient room to roost comfortably. Ensure good ventilation to prevent respiratory issues and maintain cleanliness by regularly cleaning the coop and replacing bedding.
2. **Nutrition and Water:** A balanced and nutritious diet is key to keeping your flock healthy. Provide a high-quality commercial feed specifically formulated for chickens to meet their

nutritional needs. Supplement their diet with fresh vegetables, fruits, and occasional treats, but avoid feeding them harmful or toxic foods. Additionally, always make sure your chickens have access to clean and fresh water at all times, as water is crucial for digestion and overall health.

3. **Disease Prevention and Biosecurity:** Preventing diseases is much easier than treating them, so it is crucial to implement effective biosecurity measures. Start by sourcing your chickens from reputable breeders or hatcheries to minimize the risk of introducing diseases to your flock. Quarantine new birds for at least 30 days before introducing them to the existing flock. Regularly inspect your chickens for any signs of illness, and consult a veterinarian if you notice any abnormalities. Vaccinations, proper sanitation, and good hygiene practices are also essential for disease prevention.

4. **Environmental Enrichment:** Chickens are curious and social creatures that thrive in environments that provide mental stimulation and social interaction. Consider enriching their surroundings by providing perches, dust baths, and objects for pecking and scratching. Allow them access to a secure outdoor area where they can engage in natural behaviors like foraging and dust bathing. This not only keeps them physically active but also reduces boredom and potential behavioral problems.

5. **Regular Monitoring and Health Checks:** Regularly monitoring the health of your chickens is crucial for early detection of any issues. Observe their behavior, appetite, and droppings on a daily basis. Look out for signs of illness such as lethargy, decreased appetite, abnormal feces, respiratory distress, or changes in feather condition. Conduct regular health checks by examining their eyes, beak, comb, wattles, feet, and feathers for any abnormalities. Promptly address any concerns or consult a veterinarian if necessary.

Creating a healthy and comfortable environment for your backyard flock is vital to their overall well-being and productivity. By ensuring proper housing, nutrition, disease prevention, environmental enrichment, and regular monitoring, you can keep your chickens happy, healthy, and thriving. Stay tuned for the upcoming chapters of the Chicken Health Bible, where we will delve deeper into specific aspects of chicken care, common health issues, and their treatments. Together, let's build a strong foundation for the well-being of your beloved feathered companions!

Cleaning and Disinfecting 101

Maintaining cleanliness and practicing proper disinfection techniques are crucial for creating a safe and healthy environment. Whether it's in the context of construction, day-to-day cleaning, or specific situations like poultry health, understanding the fundamentals of cleaning and disinfecting is essential. In this comprehensive guide, we will explore the various aspects of cleaning and disinfecting, starting from construction and general cleaning practices, to the art of disinfection and the safe use and disposal of disinfectants. Additionally, we will touch upon the topic of chicken health to provide a holistic understanding of maintaining cleanliness in specific contexts.

Cleaning and Disinfecting in Construction:

Construction sites often have a higher risk of dirt, dust, and debris accumulation, making proper cleaning and disinfection crucial for worker safety and the prevention of contamination. Here are some key considerations:

1. **Preparing the site:** Before construction begins, ensure the area is cleared of any existing debris or contaminants. This includes removing trash, sweeping the area, and disposing of any hazardous materials properly.
2. **Daily cleaning:** Implement a daily cleaning routine to keep the construction site tidy. This involves removing debris, sweeping or vacuuming floors, and wiping down surfaces regularly.
3. **Deep cleaning:** Conduct periodic deep cleaning sessions to eliminate stubborn stains, grime, and buildup. This may include pressure washing, scrubbing, and sanitizing surfaces, as well as steam cleaning carpets and upholstery.

The Art of Cleaning:

Cleaning is the initial step in maintaining a hygienic environment. It involves removing visible dirt, dust, and debris from surfaces. Here are some important considerations for effective cleaning:

1. **Gather the right tools:** Equip yourself with the necessary cleaning tools such as brooms, mops, vacuum cleaners, microfiber cloths, and cleaning solutions suitable for the surfaces you'll be cleaning.
2. **Follow a systematic approach:** Start by removing loose debris, then move on to dusting surfaces, wiping down with appropriate cleaners, and finishing with thorough rinsing or drying.
3. **Pay attention to high-touch areas:** Focus on frequently touched surfaces like doorknobs, light switches, countertops, and handles, as these are common breeding grounds for germs.
4. **Practice good hygiene:** Remember to wash your hands before and after cleaning to minimize the risk of cross-contamination.

How to Make a Good Disinfection:

Disinfection goes beyond cleaning and involves using chemicals or other agents to kill or inactivate pathogens, reducing the risk of infection. Here are the key steps to effective disinfection:

1. **Select the right disinfectant:** Different disinfectants target specific pathogens, so it's important to choose one that is effective against the organisms you are targeting. Look for disinfectants registered with regulatory authorities for safety and efficacy.
2. **Follow instructions:** Read and follow the manufacturer's instructions for the correct dilution ratio, contact time, and application method. Improper use may reduce effectiveness or pose health risks.
3. **Apply thoroughly:** Ensure that all surfaces and objects are adequately covered with the disinfectant solution. Pay attention to areas that are frequently touched or prone to

contamination.
4. **Allow sufficient contact time:** Most disinfectants require a certain amount of time to effectively kill pathogens. This contact time should be maintained for optimal disinfection.
5. **Ventilation and safety:** When using disinfectants, ensure proper ventilation to avoid inhaling harmful fumes. Wear appropriate personal protective equipment (PPE) such as gloves and goggles to protect yourself.

Safely Using and Disposing of Disinfectants:

Proper handling and disposal of disinfectants are essential to ensure the safety of both humans and the environment. Here are some guidelines to follow:

1. **Storage:** Store disinfectants in their original containers, away from heat and direct sunlight, and out of reach of children or pets. Clearly label containers to avoid confusion.
2. **Dilution and mixing:** Follow the manufacturer's instructions for diluting disinfectants accurately. Avoid mixing different disinfectants unless explicitly stated, as it may create harmful chemical reactions.
3. **Disposal:** Dispose of used disinfectant solutions according to local regulations. Some disinfectants can be flushed down the drain with plenty of water, while others may require specific disposal methods. Check with your local waste management authorities for guidance.
4. **Safety precautions:** Always wear appropriate PPE when handling disinfectants to prevent skin or eye irritation. If accidental exposure occurs, follow the first aid instructions provided by the manufacturer and seek medical attention if necessary.

Chicken Health Bible and Cleaning:

Maintaining cleanliness in poultry environments is crucial for preventing the spread of diseases and ensuring the well-being of the birds. Here are a few key points related to chicken health and cleaning:

1. **Biosecurity measures:** Implement strict biosecurity protocols to minimize the risk of introducing pathogens to your flock. This includes regular cleaning and disinfection of poultry houses, equipment, and tools.
2. **Proper waste management:** Dispose of poultry waste appropriately, as it can harbor disease-causing agents. Follow guidelines for composting, manure management, or disposal as per local regulations.
3. **Cleaning poultry houses:** Remove bedding, debris, and dust regularly. Clean surfaces thoroughly using appropriate cleaners and disinfectants. Pay special attention to waterers, feeders, and nesting areas.
4. **Equipment and tools:** Regularly clean and disinfect equipment and tools used in poultry farming, such as feeders, waterers, incubators, and egg trays. This helps prevent cross-contamination between batches and reduces disease transmission.

Maintaining a clean and disinfected environment is essential for promoting health, safety, and well-being. Whether in the context of construction, daily cleaning routines, or specific situations like poultry health, following proper cleaning and disinfection practices is vital. By understanding the fundamentals outlined in this guide, you can create a safe and healthy environment for yourself, your family, or your livestock, ensuring a better quality of life for all.

Providing a Healthy and Comfortable Environment

Keeping a clean and well-maintained living environment for your chickens is essential for their overall health and well-being. Regular cleaning and disinfecting not only help prevent the spread of diseases but also create a comfortable and hygienic space for your feathered friends. In this guide, we will cover the basics of cleaning and disinfecting your chicken coop, creating comfy bedding, handling outdoor runs, and managing adverse weather events to ensure the optimal health of your chickens.

Cleaning and Disinfecting the Chicken Coop:

A clean and sanitized coop is crucial to prevent the buildup of bacteria, parasites, and other harmful microorganisms. Here are some steps to follow for effective cleaning and disinfection:

1. Remove all chickens from the coop and transfer them to a temporary holding area.
2. Clear out all bedding material, droppings, and debris from the coop. Use a shovel or rake to thoroughly clean the floor, walls, and nesting boxes.
3. Wash the surfaces with a mild detergent and warm water. Scrub any stubborn stains or dirt.
4. Rinse thoroughly with clean water to remove any soap residue.
5. Allow the coop to dry completely before applying a disinfectant.
6. Choose a suitable disinfectant recommended for poultry coops and follow the manufacturer's instructions for dilution and application.
7. Apply the disinfectant to all surfaces, paying close attention to areas that are prone to contamination, such as roosts, nesting boxes, and feeders.
8. Leave the disinfectant on for the recommended contact time, usually around 10-15 minutes.
9. Rinse the coop thoroughly with clean water to remove any remaining disinfectant.
10. Allow the coop to dry completely before reintroducing the chickens.

Creating Comfy Bedding:

Comfortable bedding is essential for chickens as it provides insulation, absorbs moisture, and prevents the growth of bacteria. Follow these steps to create a cozy bedding for your chickens:

1. Choose a suitable bedding material such as straw, wood shavings, or shredded paper. Avoid using cedar shavings as they can be toxic to chickens.
2. Spread a layer of bedding material on the coop floor, ensuring a depth of at least a few inches.
3. Monitor the bedding regularly and remove any wet or soiled areas to maintain cleanliness.
4. Add fresh bedding as needed to keep the coop dry and comfortable for your chickens.

5. Consider using nesting materials, such as hay or straw, in the nesting boxes to provide a soft and clean space for egg-laying.

Handling Outdoor Runs:

If your chickens have access to an outdoor run, proper maintenance is crucial to ensure their health and safety. Here are some tips for managing outdoor runs:

1. Regularly inspect the outdoor run for any signs of damage or wear. Repair or replace any broken fencing or netting to prevent predators from entering the run.
2. Remove any debris, such as fallen branches or leaves, from the run to prevent potential hazards or hiding spots for pests.
3. Rotate the outdoor run periodically to prevent the soil from becoming compacted and contaminated with droppings.
4. Consider using movable electric netting to create temporary grazing areas for your chickens, allowing them to access fresh grass while protecting them from predators.
5. Provide access to clean water in the outdoor run to ensure hydration, especially during hot weather.

Managing Adverse Weather Events:

Extreme weather conditions can have a significant impact on your chickens' health. Here are some considerations for managing adverse weather events:

1. Extreme Heat:

A. Ensure adequate ventilation in the coop to prevent heat buildup. Install fans or vents if necessary.
B. Provide shade in the outdoor run using tarps or natural structures like trees.
C. Offer cool, fresh water at all times and consider adding electrolytes to their drinking water during heatwaves.

2. Cold Weather:

A. Insulate the coop to retain heat. Use materials like straw bales or insulation boards.
B. Ensure proper ventilation to prevent excessive moisture buildup, which can lead to respiratory issues.
C. Provide a heat source, such as a heat lamp or a heated pad, to keep the coop warm during frigid temperatures.
D. Check for drafts and seal any gaps to prevent cold air from entering the coop.

Maintaining a clean and hygienic environment for your chickens is vital for their overall health and well-being. By following proper cleaning and disinfecting practices, creating comfortable bedding, managing outdoor runs, and preparing for adverse weather events, you can ensure a healthy and comfortable living space for your feathered friends. Remember to regularly monitor and adapt your cleaning routine based on the specific needs and conditions of your chicken coop.

Keep Your Flock Fit

Keeping your flock healthy is essential for their well-being and productivity. Just like any other living creatures, chickens are susceptible to various health problems that can impact their overall fitness. In this comprehensive guide, we will discuss common health issues in chickens, major causes of death, and the importance of safely sourcing new birds. By understanding these aspects, you can ensure the health and vitality of your flock.

Common Health Problems in Chickens

1. **Respiratory Issues:** Respiratory diseases like infectious bronchitis, avian influenza, and mycoplasma infections can cause coughing, sneezing, nasal discharge, and difficulty breathing.
2. **Parasites:** External parasites like mites and lice, as well as internal parasites such as worms, can lead to feather loss, anemia, poor growth, and reduced egg production.
3. **Bacterial Infections:** Bacterial diseases like salmonella, E. coli infections, and staphylococcus infections can cause diarrhea, decreased appetite, lethargy, and even death.
4. **Viral Infections:** Viruses such as Newcastle disease and infectious bursal disease can lead to respiratory distress, diarrhea, neurological symptoms, and high mortality rates.
5. **Nutritional Deficiencies:** Poor diet or imbalanced nutrition can result in various health issues, including weak bones (osteoporosis), poor feather quality, and decreased egg production.

Major Causes of Death in Chickens

1. **Predators:** Predatory animals, such as foxes, raccoons, and hawks, can cause significant losses in a flock if proper predator-proofing measures are not in place.
2. **Disease Outbreaks:** Outbreaks of highly contagious diseases can quickly spread among a flock, leading to high mortality rates if not identified and addressed promptly.
3. **Accidents:** Accidents like getting trapped, falling from perches, or suffocating in feed containers can result in fatal injuries if appropriate safety precautions are not taken.
4. **Extreme Temperatures:** Exposure to extreme heat or cold without proper shelter or ventilation can cause heat stress, frostbite, or hypothermia, leading to death.
5. **Cannibalism and Pecking Order:** Aggressive pecking behavior or cannibalism among flock members can result in severe injuries, infections, and even death.

Safely Sourcing New Birds

1. **Biosecurity:** When introducing new birds to your flock, it is crucial to maintain strict biosecurity practices to prevent the spread of diseases. Quarantine new birds for at least two weeks to observe their health and prevent potential contagion.
2. **Reputable Sources:** Purchase birds from reputable breeders, hatcheries, or suppliers with a track record of maintaining healthy flocks and following good biosecurity measures.

3. **Physical Examination:** Inspect the new birds for signs of disease or parasites before introducing them to your existing flock. Look for healthy feathers, bright eyes, alertness, and a clean vent area.
4. **Vaccination and Testing:** Ensure that the birds have been properly vaccinated and tested for common diseases before purchasing or introducing them to your flock. This helps reduce the risk of disease transmission.
5. **Gradual Introduction:** Introduce new birds gradually, allowing them to establish their place within the pecking order. Monitor their behavior closely to prevent bullying or aggressive interactions.

Maintaining the health of your flock is of utmost importance to ensure their well-being and productivity. By familiarizing yourself with common health problems in chickens, understanding the major causes of death, and safely sourcing new birds, you can take proactive steps to keep your flock fit. Regular observation, preventive measures, and prompt veterinary care when necessary, will go a long way in keeping your chickens healthy and happy. Remember, a healthy flock is a thriving flock.

Chapter 2

Healthy Chicken Behavior

Chickens are fascinating creatures with their own unique behaviors and social dynamics. As backyard chicken keeping gains popularity, it is crucial for poultry enthusiasts and farmers alike to understand what constitutes healthy chicken behavior. In Chapter 2, we delve into the intricacies of how chickens interact, communicate, and express themselves within their flock.

This chapter serves as a comprehensive guide to deciphering the various behavioral patterns exhibited by chickens and what they signify in terms of their physical and mental well-being. We explore the significance of behaviors such as pecking order establishment, dust bathing, foraging, roosting, and vocalizations, among others.

Understanding healthy chicken behavior goes beyond mere observation; it allows us to identify signs of distress, illness, or potential problems within the flock. By equipping ourselves with this knowledge, we can take proactive measures to maintain optimal chicken health and ensure a harmonious environment for our feathered friends.

Throughout this chapter, we will delve into the instinctual behaviors chickens exhibit in response to their environment, their social hierarchy, and the roles they play within their flock. We will explore how these behaviors can be affected by factors such as breed, age, and environmental conditions.

Whether you are a novice or experienced chicken keeper, Chapter 2 will provide you with valuable insights and practical tips for promoting and maintaining healthy chicken behavior. By nurturing an environment that supports their natural instincts, you can create a thriving flock that is not only happy but also more productive in terms of egg production and overall vitality.

So, let us embark on a journey into the fascinating world of chicken behavior, where we will unravel the secrets behind their social dynamics, natural instincts, and the keys to fostering a vibrant and healthy flock.

The Chicken Daily Routine

Chickens are fascinating creatures that thrive on routine and structure. Establishing a daily routine for your flock not only promotes their overall well-being but also ensures a healthy and happy environment for them to live in. In this guide, we will explore the essential aspects of a chicken's daily routine, focusing on how to start the day, settle in for the night, and maintain a harmonious flock dynamic.

How to Start the Day:

A good morning routine sets the tone for the rest of the day and helps chickens remain active, content, and productive. Here are some key steps to consider:

1. **Early Morning Feeding:** Begin by providing fresh food and water for your flock. A balanced diet consisting of commercial poultry feed, supplemented with grains, vegetables, and occasional treats, is crucial for their health. Ensure that the feeders are clean and easily accessible.
2. **Letting Them Out:** If your chickens are housed in a coop, open the doors to allow them access to the outdoor run or free-range area. This allows them to exercise, forage for insects and plants, and soak up some natural sunlight, which is essential for their vitamin D synthesis.
3. **Daily Health Checks:** Take a few minutes to observe your chickens closely. Look for any signs of illness, injury, or abnormal behavior. Checking their feathers, skin, eyes, and droppings can give you valuable insights into their health. Address any issues promptly to prevent the spread of disease.
4. **Cleaning Duties:** Regularly clean the coop, removing soiled bedding, and replenishing it with fresh material like straw or wood shavings. Cleanliness is crucial to prevent the buildup of bacteria, parasites, and unpleasant odors.

How to Settle in for the Night:

A peaceful and secure nighttime routine is vital for chickens' rest and safety. Here's how to ensure a smooth transition from day to night:

1. **Bedtime Ritual:** As dusk approaches, chickens naturally seek a safe place to roost for the night. Make sure the coop is well-ventilated, predator-proof, and comfortable. Provide sufficient perching space, allowing each bird to have at least 8-10 inches of roosting space. Chickens prefer to sleep on elevated perches, as it helps them feel secure.
2. **Closing Up:** Close the coop door once all chickens have settled inside. This prevents predators from entering and disturbing their sleep. Ensure the coop is securely locked to safeguard against nighttime threats.
3. **Coop Security:** Regularly inspect the coop for any potential vulnerabilities. Patch up holes, reinforce latches, and fortify the structure as needed to prevent predators from gaining access. Installing motion-activated lights or alarms can provide additional security.

How to Be Together in the Flock:

Chickens are social creatures that thrive in the company of their flock mates. Encouraging a harmonious flock dynamic requires attention to their social needs:

1. **Flock Bonding:** Introduce new birds to the flock gradually, allowing them to establish a pecking order without excessive aggression. Provide sufficient space for all chickens to move around comfortably. Ensure each bird has access to food and water without being bullied.
2. **Dust Bathing:** Chickens engage in dust bathing to keep their feathers clean, control parasites, and maintain healthy skin. Provide a designated area in the coop or run, filled with dry soil or sand mixed with wood ash or diatomaceous earth. This allows them to indulge in this natural behavior.
3. **Enrichment Activities:** Stimulate your chickens' natural instincts by providing toys, perches of varying heights, and objects to peck and explore. This helps prevent boredom, reduces stress, and promotes healthy behaviors.
4. **Time in Nature:** Whenever possible, allow your flock to free-range in a safe, enclosed space or supervise them in the garden. This provides mental and physical stimulation, allowing them to engage in natural behaviors like foraging and scratching.

Remember, every flock is unique, and it may take some time to establish a routine that suits your chickens' specific needs. Observe their behavior, monitor their health, and adapt the routine as necessary to ensure a happy and thriving flock. By prioritizing their daily needs and providing a structured environment, you are contributing to their overall well-being and health.

How to Keep Peace in the flock

Keeping peace within a chicken flock is crucial for their overall well-being and productivity. Chickens, like many other animals, have a social structure that revolves around hierarchies and pecking orders. However, conflicts can arise within the flock, leading to stress, injuries, and decreased productivity. We will explore strategies to maintain harmony in the flock by understanding the role of the rooster, establishing hierarchies, and managing sibling rivalry.

The Role of the Rooster:

The presence of a rooster in the flock plays a significant role in maintaining order and peace. Roosters naturally take on the responsibility of protecting the flock from external threats and keeping the hens in line. They establish their authority by asserting dominance and mediating conflicts within the flock. The rooster's presence helps establish a sense of security, as their crowing and vigilance can deter potential predators.

Establishing Hierarchies:

Chickens have a natural inclination towards forming hierarchies, commonly referred to as the pecking order. Hierarchies help maintain order and reduce conflicts within the flock. The pecking order determines the social ranking of each chicken, with dominant individuals occupying the top positions.

1. **Providing Sufficient Space:** One way to prevent disputes and aggression is to ensure that the chickens have enough space. Overcrowding can lead to stress and territorial disputes, increasing the likelihood of aggression. Providing adequate space both inside the coop and in the outdoor run allows chickens to establish their territories and minimize conflict.
2. **Multiple Feeding Stations:** Chickens can exhibit aggressive behavior around food sources. To avoid intense competition during feeding, it is beneficial to provide multiple feeding stations spaced out throughout the flock's living area. This allows each chicken to have access to food without feeling threatened or bullied.
3. **Avoiding Sudden Introductions:** When introducing new chickens to an existing flock, it's important to do so gradually. Sudden introductions can disrupt the established hierarchy and lead to conflicts. Quarantine and supervised integration methods can help minimize aggression and allow new members to integrate more smoothly.

Managing Sibling Rivalry:

Sibling rivalry is commonly observed in flocks that include chickens from the same hatch or brood. While it is natural for young chickens to compete for resources and establish their place within the pecking order, excessive aggression can be detrimental to their well-being.

1. **Brooder Space:** Providing ample space in the brooder during the early stages of chicken development can minimize the occurrence of sibling rivalry. Sufficient room allows chicks to establish their personal space and reduces the chances of overcrowding-induced aggression.
2. **Balanced Nutrition:** Proper nutrition is crucial for promoting healthy growth and minimizing aggressive behavior. A well-balanced diet that meets the nutritional requirements of growing chicks helps reduce competition for food and may contribute to overall flock harmony.
3. **Environmental Enrichment:** Offering various forms of environmental enrichment, such as perches, toys, and hiding spots, can divert the chicks' attention and alleviate boredom. Boredom can contribute to aggressive behavior, so providing engaging environments can help reduce sibling rivalry.

Maintaining peace within a chicken flock is essential for their welfare and productivity. Understanding the role of the rooster, establishing hierarchies, and managing sibling rivalry are key elements in achieving a harmonious environment. By implementing these strategies, chicken keepers can promote the well-being of their flock, minimize stress, and create a conducive atmosphere for optimal growth and productivity. Remember, a peaceful flock is a happy flock!

How chickens communicate

Chickens, domesticated birds that have been companions to humans for thousands of years, have a unique way of communicating with each other. Their communication methods involve various vocalizations, body language, and social interactions. In this article, we will explore the different aspects of chicken communication, including the role of roosters, the chatter of hens, their interactions among themselves, and their courtship behaviors. By understanding these forms of communication, chicken owners can better care for their flock's health and well-being.

The Role of Roosters in Communication:

Roosters play a vital role in the communication dynamics within a flock. Their crowing is a well-known vocalization that serves multiple purposes. It acts as a territorial declaration, warning other roosters of their presence and asserting dominance. Roosters also use crowing as a way to announce the break of dawn, allowing hens and other chickens to synchronize their daily activities.

Apart from crowing, roosters use various calls to communicate with their hens and other members of the flock. They emit specific vocalizations to alert the flock of potential threats, such as predators or unfamiliar objects. Roosters can also produce softer, clucking sounds to indicate food discoveries, inviting the hens to join in the feeding.

The Chatter of Hens:

Hens, the female members of the chicken flock, have their unique way of communicating through vocalizations. They produce a range of clucks, purrs, and cackles, which vary in pitch and intensity. These vocalizations serve as a means of establishing social bonds, relaying information, and expressing emotions.

Hens often make distinctive vocalizations when they find food or discover a preferred nesting spot. These sounds act as a form of communication, attracting other hens to the source of interest. Additionally, hens use softer purring noises to communicate contentment and satisfaction, often observed when they are comfortable in their surroundings or after successfully laying an egg.

Talking Among Themselves:

Chickens have a complex social structure within their flocks, and they communicate extensively with each other. They use a combination of vocalizations and body language to convey messages and maintain order within the group.

Clucking sounds are common among chickens when they are engaging in casual interactions or simply going about their daily activities. Hens may emit soft clucks to indicate their approval or disapproval of a particular situation. Similarly, chickens use low growls or hisses as a warning sign, indicating aggression or discomfort.

Besides vocalizations, chickens rely on body language to communicate. Head bobbing, wing stretching, and feather fluffing are common gestures used to convey various messages. For example, a raised head accompanied by an erect comb often indicates dominance or assertiveness, whereas a lowered head may signify submission or fear.

Courtship Behaviors:

During the courtship process, chickens engage in specific behaviors to communicate their reproductive readiness and attract a mate. Roosters perform elaborate displays, including wing flapping, strutting, and puffing up their feathers. These visual signals, combined with vocalizations such as clucks and crowing, communicate the rooster's health, strength, and desirability to the hens.

Hens, on the other hand, may respond to courtship displays by displaying their receptive state through specific behaviors. This includes crouching down, spreading their wings, and making soft cooing sounds. These actions indicate that the hen is ready to mate and can be observed during the mating process.

Communication plays a crucial role in the social dynamics and overall well-being of chickens. By understanding the various vocalizations, body language, and courtship behaviors of chickens, owners can gain insights into their flock's health and ensure their welfare. Observing and interpreting these communication cues allows for better care and management practices, leading to happier and healthier chickens. The Chicken Health Bible is a comprehensive resource that can provide further guidance on the topic of chicken health, covering both communication and other aspects of caring for these remarkable birds.

Chapter 3

Biosecurity For The Backyard Flock

Biosecurity is a critical aspect of maintaining the health and well-being of your backyard flock. Implementing proper biosecurity measures helps to prevent the introduction and spread of diseases among your chickens. In Chapter 3 of the Chicken Health Bible, we will explore various aspects of biosecurity and the potential risks that can compromise the health of your flock.

How's Your Biosecurity?

Before delving into the specific risks and preventive measures, it is essential to assess the current state of your biosecurity practices. Take a moment to evaluate your biosecurity measures and identify any areas that may require improvement. Regularly reviewing and updating your biosecurity protocols will ensure that your flock remains protected.

Recognizing How Disease Is Spread in Chicken Flocks

Understanding how diseases are transmitted among chickens is crucial for implementing effective biosecurity measures. Diseases can spread through direct contact with infected birds, as well as indirect contact through contaminated objects or environments. Pathogens can be introduced into your flock through various routes, such as:

A Big Risk: The New Chicken (or the New Egg)

Introducing new chickens or eggs from external sources carries the risk of introducing diseases to your existing flock. Whenever bringing in new birds, it is important to quarantine them for a period of time to monitor their health and prevent the potential spread of diseases. Similarly, if hatching eggs or purchasing chicks, ensure that the source is reputable and disease-free.

The Other Risks: People, Other Animals, and Equipment

Humans, other animals, and equipment can inadvertently bring pathogens into your chicken environment. Visitors, including friends, family, and neighbors, should be cautious and follow biosecurity protocols when interacting with your flock. Additionally, pets and other livestock should be kept separate from your chickens to prevent the transmission of diseases. Equipment used for your flock, such as feeders, waterers, and tools, should be regularly cleaned and disinfected to minimize the risk of contamination.

Potential Critters in Chicken Feed

Chicken feed can sometimes contain unwanted visitors, such as rodents and wild birds, which can introduce diseases to your flock. Proper storage of feed in rodent-proof containers and minimizing access to wild birds can help reduce this risk. Additionally, consider using commercial feed that is specifically formulated for poultry, as it undergoes stringent quality control measures to ensure its safety.

Implementing Biosecurity Measures

To establish a robust biosecurity program for your backyard flock, consider the following preventive measures:

1. **Isolation and Quarantine:** Separate new birds from the existing flock for a quarantine period of at least 30 days. Monitor their health closely during this time and ensure they show no signs of illness before integrating them with the rest of your chickens.
2. **Sanitation Practices:** Maintain a clean and hygienic environment for your chickens. Regularly clean and disinfect coops, equipment, and any areas where chickens have access. Use appropriate disinfectants recommended for poultry use.
3. **Control Access:** Restrict access to your flock's living area. Limit the number of visitors, and ensure that anyone who comes into contact with the chickens follows proper biosecurity protocols, including hand washing and wearing clean clothes and footwear.
4. **Vermin Control:** Implement measures to control rodents and wild birds in and around the chicken area. Secure feed storage and prevent access to wild birds by using netting or covers.
5. **Disease Monitoring:** Regularly observe your flock for any signs of illness, such as changes in behavior, decreased egg production, or respiratory symptoms. Promptly isolate and seek veterinary advice if any health issues arise.

Maintaining biosecurity is essential for protecting the health and well-being of your backyard flock. By understanding how diseases are spread and implementing appropriate preventive measures, you can minimize the risk of introducing and spreading pathogens within your flock. Remember to regularly review and update your biosecurity protocols to adapt to changing circumstances and emerging disease threats. By prioritizing biosecurity, you can ensure a healthy and thriving flock of chickens.

A Biosecurity Plan

Biosecurity plays a critical role in maintaining the health and well-being of chickens. It involves a set of practices and measures aimed at preventing the introduction and spread of diseases within poultry flocks. A well-designed biosecurity plan is essential for protecting chickens from various pathogens and minimizing the risks associated with disease outbreaks. This article will explore the importance of biosecurity, discuss biosecurity habits in daily chores, and address specific considerations for show chickens.

Importance of Biosecurity:

1. **Disease Prevention:** Biosecurity measures help prevent the introduction and spread of diseases among poultry flocks. Diseases such as avian influenza, Newcastle disease, and infectious bronchitis can have devastating consequences for chicken populations.
2. **Economic Impact:** Disease outbreaks can lead to significant economic losses for poultry farmers due to increased mortality, reduced productivity, and trade restrictions.
3. **Public Health:** Some poultry diseases, such as avian influenza, can pose risks to human health. Proper biosecurity practices can reduce the potential for zoonotic transmission.

Biosecurity Habits in Daily Chores:

Developing biosecurity habits as part of your daily routine is crucial for maintaining a disease-free environment for your chickens. Here are some essential practices to incorporate:

1. **Controlled Access:** Limit access to poultry areas to authorized personnel only. Establish entry points with footbaths or sanitizing stations to prevent the introduction of contaminants.
2. **Quarantine:** Implement a quarantine period for new birds or those returning from shows or other locations. Isolate them from the existing flock for a specific duration to monitor their health status.
3. **Sanitation:** Clean and disinfect all equipment, tools, and housing regularly. Remove organic matter, such as manure and bedding, to minimize the survival of pathogens.
4. **Pest Control:** Implement measures to control pests such as rodents, wild birds, and insects, which can introduce diseases to your flock.
5. **Biosecurity Signage:** Post biosecurity signs to remind visitors and workers about the importance of adhering to biosecurity protocols.
6. **Record Keeping:** Maintain accurate records of bird movements, vaccinations, treatments, and mortalities. This information can be valuable in disease investigations.

Biosecurity for Show Chickens:

Show chickens require special considerations to ensure their health and prevent the spread of diseases within the show environment. Here are some key points to remember:

1. **Pre-Show Preparation:** Before attending a show, ensure that your birds are healthy, free

from diseases, and properly vaccinated. Consult with a veterinarian to determine the appropriate vaccination schedule.

2. **Traveling Precautions:** During transportation, provide clean and comfortable containers with adequate ventilation. Avoid contact with other birds and minimize stress levels during the journey.
3. **Isolation:** Upon returning from a show, isolate the birds from the main flock for a specific period. Monitor their health closely for any signs of illness before reintroducing them.
4. **Disinfection:** Disinfect all show equipment, such as cages, crates, and grooming tools, before and after the event. This will prevent the potential transmission of pathogens to and from other birds.
5. **Biosecurity at Shows:** Follow the biosecurity guidelines provided by the show organizers. Maintain distance between your birds and other participants, and avoid unnecessary contact with other birds and their equipment.
6. **Post-Show Evaluation:** After the show, monitor your birds for any signs of illness for an extended period. If any health issues arise, consult with a veterinarian promptly.

Implementing a robust biosecurity plan is crucial for keeping chickens healthy and minimizing the risk of disease outbreaks. By incorporating biosecurity habits into your daily chores and considering specific measures for show chickens, you can create a disease-free environment that ensures the well-being of your flock. Remember, maintaining a biosecure environment is a shared responsibility, and every poultry enthusiast should play their part in preventing the spread of diseases.

Chapter 4

Food Safety And Quality Of Homegrown Eggs And Meat

In Chapter 4 of the "Chicken Health Bible," we delve into the crucial aspects of food safety and quality when it comes to homegrown eggs and meat. Raising chickens for their eggs and meat is a rewarding endeavor, but it is vital to ensure that the food produced is safe and of high quality. This chapter provides comprehensive guidance on handling eggs, managing layers and nests, the washing debate, and proper inspection and storage techniques.

How to Properly Handle Eggs:

Eggs are highly perishable and require careful handling to maintain their freshness and prevent any contamination. In this section, we discuss the key practices for proper egg handling:

1. **Cleaning:** It is essential to clean eggs promptly to remove any dirt or debris. However, it is generally recommended to avoid washing eggs unless they are excessively soiled. Washing can remove the egg's natural protective cuticle, making it more susceptible to bacteria. Instead, dry cleaning techniques like brushing or gentle rubbing can be used for light cleaning.
2. **Collecting:** Collect eggs frequently to prevent them from sitting in the nest for extended periods. Regular collection helps minimize the risk of breakage, exposure to bacteria, and potential egg cannibalism.
3. **Handling:** Handle eggs with care to avoid cracks and fractures. Use both hands when picking up eggs to distribute the pressure evenly. Cracked eggs should not be consumed and should be discarded.
4. **Storage:** Store eggs at the right temperature to maintain their quality. It is recommended to store eggs in a cool, dark place with a consistent temperature between 40-45°F (4-7°C).

Avoid storing eggs near pungent foods as they can absorb odors.

Managing Layers and Nests:

Ensuring a clean and comfortable environment for layers and providing appropriate nest boxes are vital for producing high-quality eggs. This section highlights important factors to consider:

1. **Hygiene:** Maintaining good hygiene in the coop is crucial for egg safety. Regularly clean the nesting boxes, removing any droppings, feathers, or debris. Replace nesting materials regularly to prevent contamination.
2. **Nest Box Design:** Design nest boxes that offer privacy, comfort, and security to your hens. Provide soft bedding material like straw or shavings, ensuring it is dry and clean. Ensure adequate ventilation to prevent the accumulation of ammonia fumes.
3. **Nest Box Placement:** Place nest boxes in a quiet and dimly lit area to encourage hens to lay their eggs there. This helps prevent floor eggs and reduces the risk of contamination.
4. **Nest Egg:** To encourage hens to lay eggs in the nest boxes, consider placing fake or ceramic nest eggs. The presence of nest eggs can serve as a visual cue for hens to lay their eggs in the designated area.

To Wash or Not to Wash?

The topic of whether to wash eggs is often debated among chicken keepers. Here, we present different perspectives to help you make an informed decision:

1. **Unwashed Eggs:** Many poultry enthusiasts argue that eggs have a natural protective cuticle that prevents the entry of bacteria through the shell's pores. They believe that washing eggs removes this protective layer, making the eggs more vulnerable to contamination. Unwashed eggs can be safely stored at room temperature.
2. **Washed Eggs:** On the other hand, some argue that washing eggs with warm water and mild soap can remove potential pathogens that may be present on the shell. Washing is particularly recommended when eggs are visibly soiled. After washing, it is crucial to dry the eggs thoroughly to prevent moisture from facilitating bacterial growth.

How to Inspect and Store Eggs:

Inspecting and storing eggs correctly are key steps in ensuring food safety and maintaining egg quality. This section provides guidelines for inspection and proper storage techniques:

1. **Inspection:** Before consuming or storing eggs, inspect them for any signs of damage, such as cracks, leaks, or unusual odors. Discard any eggs that appear abnormal, as they may pose a health risk.
2. **Refrigeration:** While unwashed eggs can be stored at room temperature, refrigeration extends their shelf life. If you choose to refrigerate eggs, place them in the main body of the refrigerator, as the door shelves may be subject to temperature fluctuations. Always store eggs with the pointed end down to help maintain their freshness.

3. **Labeling:** Consider labeling eggs with the collection date to track their freshness. Use the oldest eggs first to prevent any from going to waste.
4. **Freezing:** If you have an abundance of eggs, freezing them can be a viable option. However, it is important to remove the egg from the shell and mix the yolk and white together before freezing. Raw eggs in the shell should not be frozen as they can crack due to the expansion of the liquid inside.

Chapter 4 of the "Chicken Health Bible" provides comprehensive guidance on ensuring food safety and maintaining the quality of homegrown eggs and meat. By following proper handling techniques, managing layers and nests effectively, making informed decisions about washing eggs, and implementing appropriate inspection and storage methods, you can produce safe and high-quality food for yourself and your family.

Safe High-Quality Meat from Your Own Flock

Raising your own flock of chickens provides several benefits, including access to fresh and safe high-quality meat. When you have control over the entire process, from choosing and preparing your birds to storing the meat, you can ensure the health and safety of the meat you consume. In this guide, we will take you through the steps of raising and processing chickens, ensuring that you achieve safe, high-quality meat from your own flock.

Choosing and Preparing Your Birds:

1. **Selecting the Right Breed:** Choose a breed of chicken that is known for its meat production. Popular meat chicken breeds include Cornish Cross, Freedom Rangers, and Red Rangers. Consider factors such as growth rate, feed conversion, and meat quality when selecting your birds.
2. **Housing and Nutrition:** Provide your chickens with a clean and comfortable living environment. Ensure they have access to fresh water, a balanced diet, and appropriate space to move around. A healthy and well-fed chicken will produce high-quality meat.
3. **Growth and Development:** Monitor the growth and development of your birds closely. Regularly weigh them to track their progress. A well-managed growth rate will contribute to tender and succulent meat.

How to Prepare the Work Area:

1. **Cleanliness:** Before processing your chickens, it is essential to prepare a clean and sanitized work area. Remove any clutter, debris, or potential sources of contamination. Use food-grade sanitizers to clean all surfaces and equipment.
2. **Adequate Lighting and Ventilation:** Ensure that your work area has sufficient lighting and ventilation to facilitate the processing tasks. Good lighting will help you spot any abnormalities during inspection, and proper ventilation will keep the area fresh and free from odors.

3. **Tools and Equipment:** Gather all the necessary tools and equipment required for processing chickens. This may include sharp knives, cutting boards, a plucker, a scalder (for scalding feathers), and containers for packaging and storing meat.

Sanitizing Between Birds:

1. **Prevent Cross-Contamination:** To maintain hygiene standards, sanitize your hands and any tools or surfaces that come into contact with the birds after each processing. This prevents cross-contamination and reduces the risk of foodborne illnesses.
2. **Use Food-Safe Sanitizers:** Choose sanitizers that are specifically labeled for use in food preparation areas. Follow the manufacturer's instructions for proper usage and dilution ratios.

How to Inspect Your Processed Chickens:

1. **Visual Inspection:** Examine the carcasses for any signs of disease, injury, or abnormalities. Look for healthy skin, properly formed body parts, and absence of discolored patches or foul odors.
2. **Internal Inspection:** Inspect the internal organs to ensure they are healthy and free from abnormalities. Check the liver, heart, gizzard, and intestines for any signs of disease or inflammation.
3. **Final Quality Check:** Evaluate the overall appearance and condition of the processed chicken. The meat should be firm, well-colored, and free from excessive bruising or blemishes.

Passing Judgment:

1. **Confidence in Quality:** If the inspection reveals a healthy bird with no visible issues, you can be confident that the meat is of high quality and safe for consumption.
2. **Cautionary Measures:** If you notice any abnormalities or signs of disease during inspection, exercise caution and consult a veterinarian or poultry expert for further guidance. It is important to prioritize food safety and the well-being of consumers.

Chillin' the Chicken:

1. **Cooling Process:** After processing, cool the chicken carcasses promptly to prevent bacterial growth. The optimal temperature for chilling chicken is below 40°F (4°C). Use refrigeration or ice to maintain the desired temperature.
2. **Proper Packaging:** Wrap the chilled chicken in airtight packaging, such as vacuum-sealed bags or freezer paper, to prevent freezer burn and maintain the quality of the meat during storage.

How to Prepare and Store the Meat:

1. **Proper Handling:** When cooking the chicken, follow safe handling practices, such as washing your hands, using separate cutting boards for raw and cooked meat, and cooking

the chicken to the recommended internal temperature.
2. **Freezing:** If you plan to store the meat for an extended period, freezing is the best option. Package the chicken in freezer-safe containers or bags, ensuring all air is removed to prevent freezer burn. Label each package with the date of freezing.
3. **Shelf Life:** Frozen chicken can be safely stored for several months, but for the best quality, it is recommended to consume it within 6-9 months. Always check for signs of freezer burn or spoilage before consuming frozen chicken.

By following the steps outlined in this guide, you can ensure that you produce safe, high-quality meat from your own flock of chickens. From selecting healthy birds to proper processing, inspection, and storage techniques, maintaining hygiene and food safety is paramount. Raising and processing your own chickens provides a rewarding experience, allowing you to enjoy the satisfaction of knowing the source and quality of the meat you consume.

Chapter 5

Good Nutrition For Healthy Chicken

In the world of poultry farming, one of the fundamental factors that contribute to the overall health and productivity of chickens is their nutrition. Just like humans, chickens require a balanced and nutritious diet to thrive and lead a healthy life. Chapter 5 delves into the essential aspects of good nutrition for chickens, exploring the importance of providing them with the right nutrients, understanding their dietary requirements, and implementing proper feeding practices.

This chapter serves as a comprehensive guide for both novice and experienced poultry farmers, as well as anyone interested in understanding the significance of nutrition in poultry farming. By delving into the principles of good nutrition for chickens, readers will gain valuable insights into how to optimize their flock's health, egg production, growth, and overall well-being.

The chapter begins by discussing the vital nutrients that chickens need to consume on a daily basis, such as proteins, carbohydrates, fats, vitamins, minerals, and water. Each of these nutrients plays a unique role in supporting various bodily functions, including growth, egg production, immune system function, and overall metabolism. Readers will gain a deeper understanding of the specific functions of each nutrient and their dietary sources.

Furthermore, this chapter explores the importance of providing a well-balanced diet that meets the specific nutritional requirements of chickens at different stages of their lives. From starter feeds for newly hatched chicks to grower and layer feeds for older chickens, readers will learn how to tailor their feeding regimen to ensure optimal growth, development, and egg production.

Additionally, the chapter addresses the significance of formulating and using high-quality feed. It emphasizes the importance of sourcing feed ingredients from reliable suppliers, maintaining proper storage conditions, and avoiding common pitfalls that can lead to nutrient deficiencies or imbalances.

Furthermore, alternative feed options, such as organic and non-GMO feeds, are discussed, allowing readers to make informed choices based on their specific farming practices and goals.

Finally, the chapter highlights the importance of proper feeding management and monitoring. Readers will learn about feeding schedules, portion control, and the significance of observing chickens' eating habits to detect any potential health issues or imbalances. By implementing good feeding practices, farmers can ensure that their chickens receive optimal nutrition, leading to improved overall health and productivity.

As you dive into Chapter 5, you will gain invaluable knowledge and practical tips on providing good nutrition to your chickens. By understanding their dietary needs, you will be able to create a well-balanced diet that promotes their health, vitality, and productivity, ultimately contributing to a successful and thriving poultry farming operation.

Your Chickens' Nutritional Needs

Keeping chickens healthy and thriving is a top priority for any poultry owner. Just like humans, chickens require a balanced and nutritious diet to support their growth, immune system, and overall well-being. In this article, we will explore the nutritional needs of chickens, providing you with essential information to keep your flock in top shape.

Protein:

Protein is a vital component of a chicken's diet, as it supports muscle development, feather growth, and egg production. Good sources of protein for chickens include insects, worms, legumes, and commercial poultry feeds. It is recommended to provide a balanced diet that contains around 16-20% protein for laying hens and 18-22% protein for growing chicks.

Carbohydrates:

Carbohydrates are a valuable energy source for chickens. Grains like corn, wheat, barley, and oats are excellent carbohydrate sources that should be included in their diet. Scratch grains can be given as treats but should not constitute the majority of their diet, as they are low in essential nutrients.

Fats:

Fats are a concentrated source of energy for chickens and help with the absorption of fat-soluble vitamins. Including small amounts of healthy fats in their diet, such as vegetable oil or fish oil, can be beneficial. However, it's important to avoid excessive fat intake, as it can lead to obesity and health issues.

Vitamins:

Chickens require a range of vitamins to maintain their health. Vitamin A is essential for good vision and reproductive health, while vitamin D aids in calcium absorption and bone development. B-complex vitamins play a crucial role in energy metabolism, and vitamin E supports the immune system. Providing a balanced diet with access to fresh greens, fruits, and vegetables is the best way to ensure your chickens receive an adequate supply of vitamins.

Minerals:

Minerals are necessary for strong bones, eggshell production, and overall metabolic functions. Calcium is particularly important for laying hens to prevent eggshell abnormalities. Crushed oyster shells or commercially available calcium supplements can be provided to meet their calcium needs. Other essential minerals include phosphorus, potassium, magnesium, and trace minerals like iron, zinc, and selenium.

Water:

Water is often overlooked but is a critical component of a chicken's diet. Chickens require clean and fresh water daily to stay hydrated and support essential bodily functions. Water also aids digestion and regulates body temperature. Ensure that water sources are easily accessible and clean to promote good health.

Grit:

Chickens lack teeth and require grit to help them grind and digest their food properly. Grit consists of small stones or insoluble minerals that the chickens swallow to aid in breaking down food in their gizzard. Providing a separate container of grit allows chickens to regulate their intake as needed.

Treats and Supplements:

While a balanced diet should form the foundation of your chickens' nutrition, treats and supplements can be given in moderation. Table scraps, fruits, and vegetables can be provided as occasional treats, but they should not exceed 10% of their total diet. Additionally, there are various commercially available supplements that can enhance specific aspects of your flock's health, such as probiotics for gut health or omega-3 supplements for eggs with higher nutrient content.

By understanding and meeting your chickens' nutritional needs, you can ensure their optimal health, productivity, and longevity. Remember to provide a balanced diet, fresh water, and appropriate supplements while monitoring their growth and behavior. Happy, healthy chickens will reward you with delicious eggs and delightful companionship.

Nutritional needs of different life stages

Proper nutrition is essential for the overall health and well-being of chickens at every stage of their lives. Just like humans, chickens have specific nutritional requirements that change as they progress through different life stages. Understanding and meeting these needs is crucial for maintaining optimal health, promoting growth, and maximizing productivity. In this article, we delve into the nutritional needs of chickens at various life stages, exploring key considerations outlined in the Chicken Health

Bible.

Chick Stage:

During the chick stage (0-6 weeks), chickens require a diet rich in protein and essential nutrients to support rapid growth and development. The Chicken Health Bible recommends providing a complete chick starter feed containing approximately 20-22% protein. Adequate levels of amino acids, vitamins, and minerals, such as calcium and phosphorus, are also crucial for bone and muscle development. It is essential to ensure easy access to fresh water at all times to prevent dehydration.

Grower Stage:

As chickens enter the grower stage (6-20 weeks), their dietary needs change. The Chicken Health Bible suggests transitioning from chick starter to a grower feed with a lower protein content of around 16-18%. This allows for controlled growth, preventing skeletal and metabolic issues. A balanced diet should still provide essential vitamins, minerals, and amino acids to support muscle development and feather growth. Calcium levels should be monitored and gradually increased to promote strong bone formation.

Layer Stage:

Once chickens reach the layer stage (20+ weeks), their nutritional requirements focus on egg production. The Chicken Health Bible highlights the importance of a layer feed containing approximately 16-18% protein, lower than the chick and grower stages. The diet should be enriched with calcium (around 3.5-4%) to ensure the production of strong eggshells. Adequate levels of vitamins, minerals, and omega-3 fatty acids are essential for reproductive health, feather quality, and overall vitality.

Senior Stage:

In the senior stage (beyond 2 years), chickens may experience reduced egg production and changes in metabolism. The Chicken Health Bible recommends transitioning to a maintenance or senior feed that provides balanced nutrition while supporting overall health. The feed should contain adequate levels of protein (around 16%) and essential nutrients to maintain body condition and prevent deficiencies. Adding supplements like probiotics or omega-3 fatty acids can support immune function and joint health.

Special Considerations:

In addition to the general nutritional needs of chickens at different life stages, the Chicken Health Bible highlights a few specific considerations:

1. **Molting:** During molting, chickens require additional protein and nutrients to support feather regrowth. Feeding a higher-protein molt-specific diet can aid in the molting process.
2. **Broilers:** For meat production, broiler chickens have specific nutritional requirements to promote rapid growth. High-protein feeds with an appropriate balance of essential nutrients

are necessary for achieving optimal weight gain.
3. **Free-Range Chickens:** Chickens with access to foraging areas may obtain some nutrients from natural sources. However, it is important to provide a balanced diet to ensure they receive all necessary nutrients, as foraging alone may not be sufficient.

Understanding the nutritional needs of chickens at different life stages is crucial for their health, productivity, and longevity. Following the guidelines outlined in the Chicken Health Bible regarding protein levels, essential nutrients, and special considerations ensures that chickens receive the optimal diet at each stage of their lives. By providing proper nutrition, we can support their growth, maintain strong immune systems, and ensure a healthy and productive flock.

Starter Feed/Baby Food: 0-8 Weeks

Raising healthy baby chicks requires careful attention to their nutritional needs, especially during the crucial early weeks of their lives. The right starter feed or baby food is essential for providing the necessary nutrients to support their growth and development. In this guide, we will explore the importance of a proper diet for chicks aged 0-8 weeks and provide valuable information on their nutritional requirements, with a focus on chicken health as outlined in the Chicken Health Bible.

Importance of Proper Nutrition:

Proper nutrition plays a vital role in the overall health and well-being of baby chicks. During their first few weeks of life, chicks experience rapid growth and need a diet that supplies them with essential nutrients, vitamins, and minerals. A well-balanced starter feed not only promotes healthy growth but also supports the development of strong bones, feathers, and immune systems, ensuring a solid foundation for their future as productive adult chickens.

Choosing the Right Starter Feed:

The Chicken Health Bible emphasizes the importance of selecting high-quality starter feed for optimal chick health. When choosing a starter feed, it is essential to look for specific characteristics that meet the nutritional requirements of chicks aged 0-8 weeks:

1. **Protein Content:** Chicks require a higher percentage of protein in their diet compared to adult chickens. Look for a starter feed that contains around 20-22% protein to support proper growth and muscle development.
2. **Balanced Nutrient Profile:** The starter feed should contain a balanced mix of carbohydrates, fats, vitamins, and minerals. Essential nutrients like calcium, phosphorus, and vitamin D3 are crucial for bone development and should be present in adequate amounts.
3. **Formulated for Chicks:** Opt for a starter feed specifically formulated for baby chicks, as it will be finely ground for easier digestion. Avoid using adult chicken feed, as it may lack the necessary nutrients and can be challenging for chicks to consume.

Feeding Schedule and Practices:

Establishing a consistent feeding schedule and implementing best practices are essential for the health and well-being of baby chicks:

Starter Feed Introduction:

Introduce starter feed to the chicks within the first 24-48 hours after hatching. Initially, offer small amounts of feed on a shallow dish or feeder to encourage consumption.

1. **Free Access to Feed:** Baby chicks should have access to starter feed at all times. Keep their feeders clean, dry, and easily accessible to promote healthy eating habits.
2. **Fresh Water Supply:** Alongside the starter feed, provide clean and fresh water to keep the chicks hydrated. Use shallow waterers designed specifically for chicks to prevent drowning hazards.
3. **Monitor Feed Intake:** Observe the chicks closely to ensure they are consuming an adequate amount of feed. If they appear lethargic or show signs of decreased appetite, it may indicate an underlying health issue and requires prompt attention.

Consulting the Chicken Health Bible:

The Chicken Health Bible serves as an invaluable resource for poultry owners, offering comprehensive information on various aspects of chicken health, including nutrition. It provides detailed guidelines on raising healthy chicks, managing common health issues, and optimizing the overall well-being of your flock.

Proper nutrition is crucial for the healthy growth and development of baby chicks. Following the recommendations outlined in the Chicken Health Bible, such as choosing the right starter feed, maintaining a consistent feeding schedule, and providing fresh water, will contribute to the overall health and well-being of your chicks. By prioritizing their nutritional needs during the critical 0-8 weeks period, you are setting the stage for healthy, thriving adult chickens in the future.

Grower Feed/Pullet Food: 8-16 Weeks

Providing appropriate nutrition is crucial for the healthy growth and development of chickens, particularly during their early stages. The transition from chick starter feed to grower feed, also known as pullet food, is an important milestone in the dietary needs of young chickens. In this article, we will explore the significance of grower feed for chickens aged 8 to 16 weeks, focusing on its composition, benefits, and its role in promoting overall chicken health.

The Importance of Grower Feed:

During the 8–16-week period, chickens experience significant growth and maturation. Their nutritional requirements change, necessitating a feed formulation specifically designed for their needs. Grower feed is formulated to provide balanced nutrition, helping pullets develop strong bones, robust muscles, and prepare them for egg production in the future.

Composition of Grower Feed:

Grower feed consists of a well-balanced blend of proteins, carbohydrates, fats, vitamins, and minerals. The precise composition may vary depending on the brand or manufacturer, but generally, grower feed contains approximately 16-18% protein. This protein content is slightly lower than the starter feed but higher than the layer feed meant for mature hens. Additionally, grower feed incorporates a balanced combination of grains, seeds, legumes, and other ingredients to ensure optimal growth and health.

Benefits of Grower Feed:

1. **Controlled Protein Levels:** The lower protein content in grower feed compared to starter feed helps prevent rapid growth, reducing the risk of skeletal disorders such as leg deformities or bone fractures. Controlled protein levels promote steady, healthy growth and the development of strong skeletal structure.
2. **Essential Nutrients:** Grower feed is enriched with essential vitamins and minerals required for the pullets' growth and immune system development. These nutrients include calcium, phosphorus, Vitamin D, Vitamin E, and B-complex vitamins. They support bone formation, feather growth, and overall health, reducing the likelihood of nutritional deficiencies.
3. **Optimal Energy Balance:** Pullet food is formulated to provide the right balance of carbohydrates and fats to meet the growing chickens' energy needs. This ensures steady growth and supports the development of healthy muscles and tissues.
4. **Promotes Gut Health:** Grower feed often contains probiotics or prebiotics that support a healthy gut microbiome. These beneficial microorganisms aid in digestion, absorption of nutrients, and overall gut health, reducing the risk of digestive disorders.

Feeding Recommendations:

When introducing grower feed to pullets, it's essential to follow the manufacturer's guidelines or consult with a poultry nutrition expert. Generally, it is recommended to gradually transition from starter feed to grower feed over a period of 1-2 weeks. This gradual change helps the chicks adapt to the new feed without causing digestive disturbances.

Monitor the chickens' intake and adjust the quantity as necessary to prevent overeating or wastage. Ensure a constant supply of clean, fresh water alongside grower feed, as adequate hydration is vital for their health and digestion.

Providing appropriate nutrition during the 8–16-week stage is crucial for the long-term health and productivity of chickens. Grower feed offers a balanced and tailored blend of nutrients that support steady growth, strong bone development, and overall well-being. By feeding pullets with the right nutrition during this critical period, you are laying the foundation for healthy, thriving chickens that will go on to provide years of egg-laying happiness in the future.

Layer Feed for Hens: 16 Weeks and Up

As backyard chicken enthusiasts, it is essential to provide our feathered friends with a balanced and nutritious diet to promote their health and productivity. Once your hens reach 16 weeks of age, they are considered mature and ready to transition to a specialized diet known as layer feed. In this article, we will delve into the importance of layer feed, its composition, and the benefits it offers to your flock's overall well-being. This information is an excerpt from the comprehensive resource, the Chicken Health Bible, designed to help you raise healthy and happy chickens.

Understanding Layer Feed:

Layer feed is specifically formulated to meet the nutritional requirements of laying hens. It provides a well-balanced combination of essential nutrients, including proteins, carbohydrates, vitamins, and minerals, necessary for egg production and maintaining hen health. This specialized feed ensures that your hens receive the specific nutrients they need to produce high-quality eggs and sustain their overall well-being.

Composition of Layer Feed:

Layer feed typically consists of a mix of various ingredients, each serving a specific purpose. Here are some common components found in layer feed:

1. **Protein sources:** Layer feed contains high-quality protein sources such as soybean meal, fish meal, and grains. Protein is essential for egg production, feather health, and overall growth and repair of tissues.
2. **Calcium:** Adequate calcium is crucial for the development of strong eggshells. Layer feed incorporates calcium sources like limestone, oyster shells, or ground eggshells, ensuring hens receive the necessary calcium levels for healthy egg production.
3. **Grains and carbohydrates:** Grains like corn, wheat, and barley are included in layer feed to provide energy for your hens. Carbohydrates derived from grains are an important energy source for their daily activities.
4. **Essential vitamins and minerals:** Layer feed is fortified with vitamins and minerals like vitamin A, vitamin D, vitamin E, and various B vitamins. These nutrients support overall health, immunity, and optimal egg production.

Benefits of Layer Feed:

By providing layer feed to your mature hens, you offer several benefits that contribute to their well-being and productivity:

1. **Enhanced egg quality:** Layer feed ensures that hens receive the necessary nutrients to produce eggs with strong, consistent shells and vibrant yolks rich in nutrients.
2. **Optimal egg production:** The balanced nutritional profile of layer feed promotes consistent egg-laying, supporting higher production rates throughout the year.
3. **Improved hen health:** Layer feed contains essential vitamins and minerals that bolster the

immune system, reducing the risk of diseases and ensuring your hens remain healthy and active.

4. **Balanced nutrition:** By feeding your hens with layer feed, you can be confident that they are receiving a complete and balanced diet, reducing the need for additional supplements.

Feeding Recommendations:

To ensure your hens receive the right amount of layer feed, consider the following recommendations:

1. **Provide free access to feed:** Allow your hens to have continuous access to layer feed. They will self-regulate their intake based on their nutritional needs.
2. **Monitor feed consumption:** Keep an eye on how much feed your hens consume on average each day. This will help you gauge their nutritional requirements and detect any sudden changes in appetite that may indicate health issues.
3. **Offer fresh water:** Always provide fresh, clean water alongside layer feed. Hens need an adequate water supply to digest and utilize the nutrients from their feed effectively.

Feeding your mature hens with a high-quality layer feed is crucial for their health, egg production, and overall well-being. The carefully formulated nutritional profile of layer feed ensures that your hens receive the necessary nutrients to lay strong, nutritious eggs consistently. By following the recommendations outlined in the Chicken Health Bible, you can ensure your flock's dietary needs are met, resulting in healthy, productive hens that bring joy and delicious eggs to your backyard.

The Importance of Grit

When it comes to raising chickens, ensuring their health and well-being is of utmost importance. However, the journey of chicken farming can be fraught with challenges and obstacles that can put their health at risk. To navigate these challenges successfully, one quality that every chicken farmer should possess is grit.

Grit, in the context of chicken farming, refers to the perseverance and passion to overcome difficulties and achieve long-term goals. It is the ability to stay committed, determined, and resilient in the face of adversity. Building grit is essential for ensuring the health and well-being of your flock, as it enables you to tackle various issues head-on and find effective solutions. Here are some reasons why grit is crucial in the realm of chicken health:

Disease Prevention:

Raising healthy chickens involves implementing preventive measures to minimize the risk of diseases. However, even with careful planning, outbreaks can occur. Grit allows you to confront and combat diseases by taking prompt action. It helps you stay determined in implementing biosecurity measures, such as regular sanitization, quarantine protocols, and vaccinations, reducing the likelihood of illness spreading through your flock.

Emergency Response:

Chicken farming is vulnerable to unexpected emergencies, such as extreme weather events or predator attacks. These situations can be distressing and require immediate action to protect your flock. Grit ensures that you remain composed, think on your feet, and swiftly address the situation to minimize harm to your chickens. It empowers you to take necessary steps like reinforcing coops, securing enclosures, or providing emergency medical care, thus safeguarding the health of your birds.

Problem Solving:

Chicken health issues can be complex, and finding solutions may require critical thinking and troubleshooting. Grit helps you persevere through challenges, such as identifying the cause of an illness, devising a treatment plan, or adjusting the diet to address nutritional deficiencies. It enables you to seek expert advice, conduct research, and experiment with different strategies until you find the most effective solution for maintaining the health of your flock.

Adaptability:

The world of chicken farming is constantly evolving, with new diseases, management practices, and technologies emerging. To ensure the health of your chickens, it is essential to stay updated and adapt to these changes. Grit allows you to embrace innovation, learn new skills, and implement improved techniques for disease prevention, biosecurity, and overall flock management. By staying adaptable, you can proactively respond to emerging challenges and provide the best possible care for your chickens.

Emotional Resilience:

Raising chickens can be emotionally demanding, especially when faced with setbacks or losses. Grit helps you maintain emotional resilience by acknowledging the difficulties but not letting them deter you from your long-term goals. It allows you to bounce back from setbacks, learn from mistakes, and stay motivated to provide optimal care for your flock. Emotional resilience is essential for maintaining a positive mindset and ensuring that your own well-being does not compromise the health of your chickens.

The importance of grit in the realm of chicken health cannot be overstated. It empowers you as a chicken farmer to navigate challenges, take decisive action, and find effective solutions to protect the well-being of your flock. By embracing grit, you build resilience, adaptability, and emotional strength, enabling you to overcome obstacles and create a healthy and thriving chicken farm. So, cultivate grit in your chicken farming journey and witness the positive impact it has on the health and happiness of your feathered friends.

Grains & Goodies

Welcome to Grains & Goodies, your one-stop destination for all things related to chicken health and nutrition. In this article, we will delve into the essential aspects of maintaining your chickens' well-being while focusing on the topic of the "Chicken Health Bible." Specifically, we will explore the role of grains and other nutritious goodies in ensuring your chickens lead a healthy and vibrant life.

Chickens are incredible creatures that provide us with fresh eggs, flavorful meat, and delightful companionship. Just like humans, these feathered friends require a balanced diet to thrive. While commercial feeds are readily available, supplementing their diet with grains and other goodies can significantly enhance their overall health.

Grains, such as corn, wheat, barley, and oats, are excellent sources of energy for chickens. They are rich in carbohydrates, which provide the necessary fuel for their daily activities. Incorporating grains into their diet helps maintain their energy levels, supports proper growth, and assists in maintaining a healthy body weight.

When it comes to the Chicken Health Bible, grains play a crucial role in providing essential nutrients. They contain B vitamins, including thiamine, riboflavin, and niacin, which are vital for overall health and metabolism. These vitamins contribute to the proper functioning of the nervous system, aid in digestion, and support healthy feather development.

In addition to grains, including other goodies in your chickens' diet can be beneficial. Let's explore a few options:

1. **Legumes:** Legumes like soybeans, lentils, and peas are excellent sources of protein. Protein is essential for muscle development, egg production, and overall growth. By including legumes in their diet, you can ensure your chickens receive a well-rounded protein intake.
2. **Fresh Fruits and Vegetables:** Just like humans, chickens can benefit from a variety of fresh fruits and vegetables. These provide a range of vitamins, minerals, and antioxidants that support their immune system and overall health. Some suitable options include leafy greens, carrots, pumpkins, apples, and berries.
3. **Calcium Sources:** Calcium is vital for eggshell formation and skeletal health in chickens. Including calcium-rich sources like crushed oyster shells or ground eggshells in their diet can help prevent calcium deficiencies and promote strong egg production.
4. **Kitchen Scraps:** Instead of throwing away your kitchen scraps, consider sharing them with your chickens. While certain foods like onions, garlic, and citrus should be avoided, vegetable peels, bread crusts, and leftover rice or pasta can be great additions to their diet, reducing waste while providing extra nutrients.

Remember, a balanced diet is key to maintaining your chickens' health. Whole grains and goodies can enhance their nutrition, they should be offered in moderation and alongside a quality commercial feed specifically formulated for chickens.

Observing your chickens' behavior and consulting the Chicken Health Bible will help you understand their dietary needs better. Ensure they have access to fresh water at all times and provide a clean and spacious environment to keep them happy and healthy.

At Grains & Goodies, we believe that a well-nourished chicken is a happy chicken. By incorporating grains and other nutritious goodies into their diet, you can contribute to their overall health, longevity, and enjoyment of life. Remember, healthy chickens make for productive and contented companions.

What Not to Feed

Keeping chickens as pets or for egg production can be a rewarding experience. To ensure their health and well-being, it's important to provide them with a balanced diet. While chickens are omnivores and can eat a wide variety of foods, there are certain items that should never be fed to them. In this guide, we will explore what not to feed your chickens to maintain their optimal health.

Processed Foods:

Chickens should never be fed processed foods that are high in salt, sugar, additives, or preservatives. These include chips, cookies, candy, fast food, and any other human junk food. Such foods can be detrimental to their overall health, leading to obesity, digestive issues, and reduced egg production.

Toxic Plants:

Some plants are toxic to chickens and should be avoided at all costs. These include but are not limited to, nightshade plants (such as tomatoes, potatoes, and eggplant), rhubarb leaves, azaleas, oleander, and yew. Consuming these plants can cause various health problems ranging from gastrointestinal issues to organ failure and even death.

Avocado:

Avocado flesh and pit contain a substance called persin, which is toxic to chickens. It can cause respiratory distress, heart failure, and even death. Avoid feeding chickens any part of the avocado to ensure their well-being.

Chocolate and Caffeine:

Chocolate contains theobromine, a compound that can be toxic to chickens. Consumption of chocolate can lead to abnormal heart rhythms, seizures, and even death. Similarly, caffeine found in coffee, tea, and energy drinks can have adverse effects on their health. Avoid exposing chickens to these substances.

Onions and Garlic:

Onions and garlic, when ingested in large quantities, can cause anemia in chickens. They contain compounds that can damage red blood cells, leading to a reduced ability to carry oxygen. While small amounts may not cause harm, it's best to avoid feeding these foods to chickens altogether.

Citrus Fruits:

Citrus fruits, such as oranges, lemons, and grapefruits, should be given in moderation or avoided. The acidity of these fruits can disrupt the pH balance in a chicken's digestive system, leading to digestive upset or even diarrhea. Introduce citrus fruits gradually and observe your chickens' response.

Raw Beans:

Raw or undercooked beans, including kidney beans, can contain a toxin called lectin. Chickens are unable to digest this toxin properly, which can result in severe gastrointestinal distress and even death. Always cook beans thoroughly before feeding them to chickens.

While chickens are known for their ability to consume a wide variety of foods, it's crucial to be aware of what not to feed them. Avoid processed foods, toxic plants, avocado, chocolate, caffeine, onions, garlic, raw beans, and excessive citrus fruits to maintain their health and well-being. By providing a balanced diet and avoiding harmful foods, you can ensure that your chickens lead a happy and healthy life. Remember, when in doubt, consult with a veterinarian specializing in poultry care for specific dietary guidelines.

Carbohydrates

In the pursuit of maintaining optimal health for chickens, it is crucial to pay attention to their nutritional needs. While proteins and fats often take center stage in discussions about chicken diets, carbohydrates also play a significant role in providing the energy and essential nutrients that chickens require. This article delves into the importance of carbohydrates in the context of the Chicken Health Bible, highlighting their functions, sources, and benefits.

Understanding Carbohydrates:

Carbohydrates are one of the three main macronutrients, alongside proteins and fats. They are organic compounds composed of carbon, hydrogen, and oxygen. In the chicken's body, carbohydrates serve as a primary source of energy. When consumed, they are broken down into glucose, which fuels various physiological processes.

Functions of Carbohydrates:

1. **Energy Production:** Carbohydrates are the preferred energy source for chickens. Glucose obtained from carbohydrates is readily used by cells to fuel essential functions, such as muscle contractions, organ function, and egg production.
2. **Body Heat Regulation:** Chickens require sufficient carbohydrates to regulate their body temperature. During colder weather, carbohydrates are metabolized to generate heat through thermogenesis, helping chickens maintain their body warmth.
3. **Nutrient Storage:** Carbohydrates are stored in the form of glycogen in the chicken's liver and muscles. This stored glycogen can be rapidly converted back into glucose when the

bird requires quick energy.

Sources of Carbohydrates:

1. **Grains:** Various grains, such as corn, wheat, barley, and oats, are excellent sources of carbohydrates for chickens. These grains can be incorporated into their diet in the form of whole grains or as part of balanced poultry feeds.
2. **Fruits and Vegetables:** Fruits like apples, berries, and melons, and vegetables such as carrots, sweet potatoes, and leafy greens, provide carbohydrates along with essential vitamins and minerals. These can be offered as treats or included in the overall diet.
3. **Legumes:** Legumes like peas, lentils, and beans are not only rich in protein but also contain carbohydrates. Including legumes in the chicken's diet provides a balanced nutrient profile.

Benefits of Carbohydrates in Chicken Diets:

1. **Sustained Energy:** Carbohydrates provide a steady and sustained release of energy, ensuring chickens have the stamina to perform physical activities, forage, and lay eggs consistently.
2. **Improved Digestive Health:** Carbohydrates, particularly those derived from dietary fiber, support healthy digestion in chickens. They aid in maintaining a well-functioning gut, promoting nutrient absorption, and preventing digestive disorders.
3. **Optimal Growth and Development:** Adequate carbohydrate intake is vital for growing chicks. It supports the development of muscles, bones, and vital organs, ensuring they reach their full potential.
4. **Egg Production:** Carbohydrates play a crucial role in sustaining egg production in laying hens. Sufficient carbohydrate intake helps maintain a consistent supply of energy needed for ovulation and the production of high-quality eggs.

In the realm of the Chicken Health Bible, carbohydrates hold a prominent place in providing the energy, nutrients, and overall health benefits that chickens require. By incorporating a balanced diet that includes adequate carbohydrate sources, poultry owners can help their chickens maintain optimal health, support growth and development, and ensure steady egg production. Remember, a well-rounded diet encompassing proteins, fats, and carbohydrates is key to raising healthy and thriving chickens.

Fats

In the Chicken Health Bible, an essential aspect of poultry nutrition that cannot be overlooked is the role of fats. While fats have often been demonized in human diets, they play a crucial role in the overall health and well-being of chickens. Understanding the importance of fats and their appropriate inclusion in chicken diets is essential for maintaining optimal health, growth, and production in poultry.

Energy Source:

Fats are a highly concentrated source of energy for chickens. They provide more than twice the amount of energy compared to proteins and carbohydrates. This energy is essential for chickens to perform various physiological functions, including maintaining body temperature, growth, and egg production. Including appropriate levels of fats in the diet ensures that chickens have the energy reserves required to meet their metabolic needs.

Nutrient Absorption:

Certain vitamins, such as vitamins A, D, E, and K, are fat-soluble, which means they require the presence of dietary fats for proper absorption. These vitamins play vital roles in the immune system, bone health, and overall growth of chickens. By including fats in the diet, poultry owners can ensure that their chickens are able to absorb and utilize these essential nutrients effectively.

Essential Fatty Acids:

Fats also provide essential fatty acids that chickens cannot produce on their own. Omega-3 and omega-6 fatty acids are two examples of these essential fats. These fatty acids are necessary for the normal development and functioning of various body systems, including the immune system, nervous system, and reproductive system. By incorporating appropriate sources of essential fatty acids in the diet, such as fish oil or flaxseed, chicken owners can promote optimal health and disease resistance in their flock.

Feather Quality:

Fats contribute to the development of healthy feathers in chickens. Feathers are primarily composed of protein, but the presence of fats is essential for proper feather growth and maintenance. Adequate fat intake ensures that chickens can produce feathers that are strong, flexible, and resistant to damage. Healthy feathers not only protect chickens from environmental stressors but also contribute to their overall appearance and vitality.

Palatability and Diet Formulation:

Including fats in the diet enhances palatability, making it more likely that chickens will consume a balanced diet. This is particularly important when formulating diets for chicks or during periods of stress or illness when chickens may have decreased appetite. By using fats judiciously, poultry owners can improve the acceptance and consumption of essential nutrients, supporting the overall health and well-being of their flock.

In the Chicken Health Bible, understanding the role of fats is essential for optimizing the health and performance of chickens. Fats provide a concentrated source of energy, aid in the absorption of fat-soluble vitamins, supply essential fatty acids, contribute to feather quality, and enhance diet palatability. By carefully considering the inclusion of fats in the diet and selecting appropriate sources, poultry owners can promote the overall well-being and productivity of their chickens.

Proteins

In the vast world of nutrition, proteins hold a crucial place, particularly when it comes to the health and well-being of chickens. Proteins are essential macronutrients made up of amino acids, which are the building blocks of life. Just like humans, chickens require a sufficient intake of proteins to thrive, grow, and maintain optimal health. In this chapter of the Chicken Health Bible, we delve into the importance of proteins for these feathered creatures and explore how they contribute to their overall well-being.

Essential for Growth and Development:

Proteins play a vital role in the growth and development of chickens. From the moment a chick emerges from its shell, proteins are necessary for the formation and repair of cells, tissues, and organs. The amino acids derived from proteins are instrumental in building strong muscles, promoting bone development, and ensuring proper organ function. They act as the backbone of the chicken's physiological structure, enabling it to flourish into a healthy and robust bird.

Of Bodily Functions:

Proteins are involved in various physiological processes that are crucial for a chicken's everyday functions. Enzymes, which are specialized proteins, facilitate biochemical reactions within the body, such as digestion, metabolism, and nutrient absorption. Proteins also form antibodies, which are essential for the chicken's immune system, protecting it from harmful pathogens and diseases. Additionally, proteins are responsible for transporting vital substances, such as oxygen, across the body, ensuring the proper functioning of different organs and systems.

Source of Energy:

While carbohydrates and fats are typically the primary sources of energy for chickens, proteins also contribute to meeting their energy needs. When the body's carbohydrate and fat reserves are depleted, proteins can be broken down into amino acids and converted into energy through a process called gluconeogenesis. However, it's important to note that relying on proteins as an energy source is not ideal for chickens, as it can hinder their growth and negatively impact their overall health.

1. **Feeding the Feathered Appetite:** The diet of a chicken must provide a sufficient amount of high-quality proteins to meet its nutritional requirements. Good sources of protein for chickens include animal-based proteins like insects, worms, and fishmeal, as well as plant-based proteins such as soybean meal and peas. A well-balanced diet should contain a proper balance of essential amino acids to support the chicken's growth, reproduction, and overall vitality. Ensuring that chickens receive an adequate protein intake is crucial for maintaining their health and productivity.
2. **Protein Deficiency and Excess:** Both protein deficiency and excess can have detrimental effects on a chicken's health. Inadequate protein intake can lead to stunted growth, weakened immune system, reduced egg production, and poor muscle development.

Conversely, excessive protein consumption can strain the kidneys, leading to renal damage and increased water consumption. Achieving the right balance is key to keeping chickens healthy and thriving.

Proteins are the fundamental building blocks of chicken health. From supporting growth and development to maintaining bodily functions and providing energy, proteins play a crucial role in the overall well-being of these birds. By ensuring that chickens receive a well-balanced diet that includes adequate and high-quality proteins, chicken owners can promote their health, productivity, and longevity. Remember, when it comes to chicken health, proteins are an indispensable part of the equation.

Vitamins & Minerals

Proper nutrition plays a vital role in maintaining the health and well-being of chickens. Among the many essential components of a balanced diet, vitamins and minerals are critical for supporting various bodily functions, promoting growth, and enhancing immune response. In this article, we explore the importance of vitamins and minerals in the context of chicken health, emphasizing their role in maintaining optimal well-being and productivity. Whether you are a backyard chicken keeper or a commercial poultry farmer, understanding the significance of these essential elements is crucial for the overall health of your flock.

Vitamins:

The Key to Vitality Vitamins are organic compounds that are required in small quantities but play a significant role in the overall health and development of chickens. They serve as cofactors for numerous enzymatic reactions, helping regulate various bodily functions. Here are some essential vitamins for chickens:

1. **Vitamin A:** This vitamin is crucial for maintaining healthy vision, promoting growth, and supporting the immune system. It is commonly found in green leafy vegetables, carrots, and eggs.
2. **Vitamin D:** Essential for proper calcium absorption, vitamin D ensures strong bones and eggshell formation. Chickens can synthesize vitamin D when exposed to sunlight, but supplementation is necessary in areas with limited sunlight.
3. **Vitamin E:** As a potent antioxidant, vitamin E helps protect cells from damage, supports immune function, and enhances fertility. Good sources of vitamin E include wheat germ, sunflower seeds, and green vegetables.
4. **Vitamin K:** Required for blood clotting and bone metabolism, vitamin K is vital for maintaining healthy chickens. It is found in green leafy vegetables, alfalfa, and soybean meal.

Minerals:

Building Blocks of Health Minerals are inorganic substances that chickens require in small quantities for various physiological functions. They contribute to skeletal structure, muscle function, enzyme activity, and electrolyte balance. Some essential minerals for chickens include:

1. **Calcium:** Crucial for bone development, muscle contraction, and eggshell formation, calcium is a fundamental mineral for chickens. Sources include limestone, oyster shell, and crushed eggshells.
2. **Phosphorus:** Working in conjunction with calcium, phosphorus supports bone development and energy metabolism. It can be obtained from meat and bone meal, fishmeal, and grains.
3. **Iron:** Required for red blood cell formation and oxygen transport, iron plays a vital role in overall chicken health. Green leafy vegetables, meat, and poultry by-products are good sources of iron.
4. **Zinc:** Important for growth, feather development, and immune function, zinc is an essential mineral for chickens. It can be found in seafood, whole grains, and legumes.

Vitamins and minerals are essential elements in maintaining optimal health and productivity in chickens. Providing a well-balanced diet that includes a variety of vitamin-rich foods and mineral supplements is crucial for supporting their growth, immune response, and overall well-being. Proper nutrition ensures strong bones, healthy feathers, improved egg production, and robust immune systems, leading to thriving and resilient flocks. Remember, consulting with a poultry nutritionist or veterinarian can help tailor the diet to the specific needs of your chickens, ensuring they receive the right balance of vitamins and minerals for optimal health.

Water

In the world of poultry farming, maintaining optimal chicken health is of utmost importance. Along with providing proper nutrition and a comfortable environment, ensuring access to clean and fresh water is essential for the well-being of your flock. In this chapter of the Chicken Health Bible, we delve into the significance of water and its role in promoting the overall health and productivity of chickens.

Hydration and Body Functions:

Water is a fundamental component of every living organism, and chickens are no exception. Adequate hydration is essential for the proper functioning of a chicken's body systems, including digestion, metabolism, circulation, and temperature regulation. Water helps transport nutrients, eliminate waste products, and maintain electrolyte balance within the bird's body. Without sufficient water intake, chickens can become dehydrated, leading to various health issues.

Nutrient Absorption:

Water plays a crucial role in facilitating nutrient absorption in chickens. Many vital nutrients, such as proteins, carbohydrates, vitamins, and minerals, are transported through the bloodstream and dissolved in water. By drinking sufficient amounts of water, chickens optimize their ability to absorb these essential nutrients, supporting their growth, development, and immune function.

Digestion and Gut Health:

Proper hydration is essential for optimal digestion in chickens. Water helps soften food and aids in the breakdown of feed particles, making it easier for the digestive system to process nutrients. Additionally, water assists in the movement of food through the digestive tract, preventing constipation and promoting regular bowel movements. Maintaining a healthy gut is crucial for chickens to absorb nutrients effectively and prevent digestive disorders.

Temperature Regulation:

Chickens do not have sweat glands and rely on other mechanisms to regulate their body temperature. Water is instrumental in this process. Chickens often consume more water during hot weather as it helps them cool down through evaporative cooling. By drinking water, chickens are better equipped to cope with heat stress and maintain their body temperature within a healthy range.

Immune System Support:

Adequate water intake is closely linked to a robust immune system in chickens. Water helps flush out toxins and waste products from the body, allowing the immune system to function optimally. Additionally, water helps maintain mucous membranes in the respiratory and digestive tracts, acting as a protective barrier against pathogens. By providing clean and fresh water, you enhance your chickens' immune response, reducing the risk of disease and improving overall flock health.

Water is a critical component of the Chicken Health Bible. By recognizing the importance of proper hydration, poultry farmers can significantly contribute to the well-being, growth, and productivity of their flocks. Regular access to clean and fresh water ensures optimal digestion, nutrient absorption, temperature regulation, and immune system support in chickens. As a responsible poultry farmer, prioritize water management as an integral part of your overall flock health strategy, and your chickens will thrive.

Chapter 6

Anatomy And Body Functions

Welcome to Chapter 6 of the Chicken Health Bible! In this chapter, we will delve into the fascinating world of chicken anatomy and body functions. Understanding the intricate structures and processes that make up a chicken's body is crucial for every poultry owner or enthusiast. By familiarizing ourselves with the inner workings of these incredible creatures, we can better comprehend their health needs and provide them with optimal care.

This chapter will take you on a journey through the various systems and organs that enable a chicken to function effectively. We will explore the skeletal system, which provides support and protection, and the muscular system, responsible for movement and coordination. We will also delve into the digestive system, which plays a vital role in processing food and extracting nutrients.

Furthermore, we will examine the respiratory system, which facilitates breathing and oxygen exchange, and the circulatory system, responsible for transporting nutrients, hormones, and oxygen throughout the body. The nervous system, essential for coordinating bodily functions and responding to external stimuli, will also be discussed.

Additionally, we will explore the reproductive system, shedding light on the intricacies of egg production and the process of mating. We will uncover the secrets of the immune system, which defends against diseases and keeps our feathered friends healthy. Lastly, we will touch upon the endocrine system, which regulates various bodily functions through the release of hormones.

Throughout this chapter, we will provide detailed information on the structure and functions of each system, highlighting key considerations for maintaining optimal chicken health. By the end, you will have a comprehensive understanding of how a chicken's body operates and how to identify potential health issues.

Whether you are a backyard chicken keeper or a commercial poultry farmer, this chapter will equip you with the knowledge necessary to ensure the well-being of your feathered companions. Remember, a strong grasp of chicken anatomy and body functions is the foundation of good poultry care, enabling you to detect and address health concerns promptly.

So, let's embark on this enlightening exploration of chicken anatomy and body functions, and discover the wonders that lie beneath those beautiful feathers!

Eyes, ears, skin, and feathers

When it comes to ensuring the well-being of our feathered friends, chickens, understanding the various aspects of their health is crucial. Among these aspects are the eyes, ears, skin, and feathers. Each plays a significant role in a chicken's overall health and requires attention and care. In this article, we will delve into these vital components of chicken health, exploring their functions, common problems, and best practices for maintaining their optimal condition.

1. **Eyes:** The eyes are a chicken's window to the world. They allow chickens to navigate their surroundings and detect potential threats or opportunities. Keeping a close eye on your chickens' eyes is vital for early detection of any issues. Common eye problems in chickens include infections, conjunctivitis, and injuries. Signs of eye problems may include redness, swelling, discharge, or difficulty in opening or closing the eyes. Consultation with a veterinarian is recommended for accurate diagnosis and appropriate treatment.

To promote healthy eyes in chickens, ensure adequate lighting in their coop, protect them from dust and debris, and regularly clean their living environment. Additionally, a balanced diet rich in vitamin A is essential for good eye health.

2. **Ears:** While chickens don't rely heavily on their hearing, their ears still play a role in detecting danger and maintaining balance. Ear infections or mites can lead to discomfort and affect a chicken's overall well-being. Symptoms of ear problems may include head shaking, scratching, or abnormal behavior. A veterinarian can help diagnose and treat any ear-related issues.

To keep chicken ears healthy, maintain a clean coop, free from excessive noise or loud machinery. Regularly inspect their ears for signs of irritation or mites, and take appropriate measures to address any concerns promptly.

3. **Skin**: The skin is the largest organ in a chicken's body, and it serves as a barrier against pathogens and environmental factors. Healthy skin is crucial for protecting chickens from infections and parasites. Common skin issues in chickens include mites, lice, fungal infections, and wounds.

Regularly inspect your chickens' skin, paying close attention to featherless or bare patches, redness, swelling, or signs of irritation. Maintain a clean coop, provide dust baths, and practice good biosecurity measures to prevent and control skin problems. Consult with a veterinarian for accurate diagnosis and appropriate treatment if any issues arise.

4. **Feathers:** Feathers are not just beautiful adornments but also serve various essential functions for chickens. They provide insulation, protect against weather elements, assist in

communication, and aid in flight. Maintaining healthy feathers is crucial for a chicken's well-being.

To promote healthy feather growth, provide a balanced diet rich in essential nutrients, including protein and amino acids. Ensure chickens have access to dust baths, which help keep their feathers clean and aid in the removal of parasites. Regularly inspect feathers for signs of mites, lice, or damage. If feather problems persist or worsen, seek veterinary advice.

The eyes, ears, skin, and feathers of chickens are integral components of their overall health. Regular observation, early detection of problems, and prompt intervention are essential for maintaining these aspects in optimal condition. By prioritizing the well-being of these vital components, chicken owners can help ensure their feathered friends live a healthy and happy life. Remember, consulting with a veterinarian is always recommended when dealing with specific health concerns or issues related to eyes, ears, skin, or feathers in chickens.

Breathing and circulating blood

In the vast world of poultry health, understanding the intricate processes of breathing and circulating blood is of utmost importance. Just like any living creature, chickens rely on these vital functions to maintain their well-being. In this article, we will explore the significance of breathing and circulating blood in the context of chicken health and provide insights into how to ensure these processes run smoothly for optimal poultry care.

Breathing, a fundamental function shared by all living organisms, plays a critical role in supplying oxygen to the cells and removing carbon dioxide. Chickens have a unique respiratory system that differs from mammals, and comprehending its nuances is essential for maintaining their health. Unlike humans, chickens lack a diaphragm, which means they rely on the expansion and contraction of their ribcage to facilitate breathing.

The process of breathing in chickens begins with the inhalation of air through the nostrils. As the air enters the nasal cavity, it passes over mucus-covered surfaces, where dust and other particulate matter are trapped. The air then moves down the trachea and into the syrinx, a specialized vocal organ unique to birds. From the syrinx, the air proceeds to the bronchi, which branch out into smaller tubes called bronchioles. These bronchioles eventually terminate in tiny air sacs known as avian lungs, where gas exchange takes place.

Proper ventilation is crucial for maintaining respiratory health in chickens. Ammonia buildup from poorly ventilated chicken coops can lead to respiratory issues, such as respiratory distress syndrome or infectious bronchitis. Adequate airflow and regular cleaning of the coop are essential to prevent these respiratory ailments. Additionally, minimizing exposure to airborne pathogens, such as bacteria and viruses, is crucial for maintaining a healthy respiratory system in chickens.

While breathing ensures the intake of oxygen, the process of circulating blood ensures the delivery of oxygen and vital nutrients throughout a chicken's body. Chickens have a closed circulatory system, meaning their blood is contained within a network of vessels. The heart, a vital organ, is responsible for pumping oxygenated blood to the body and returning deoxygenated blood back to the lungs.

A chicken's heart consists of four chambers: two atria and two ventricles. The atria receive blood returning to the heart, while the ventricles pump blood out of the heart. Deoxygenated blood from the body enters the right atrium, moves into the right ventricle, and is then pumped to the lungs via the pulmonary artery. In the lungs, oxygen is absorbed, and carbon dioxide is released. Oxygenated blood returns to the heart via the pulmonary veins and enters the left atrium. It is then pumped into the left ventricle, which sends the oxygenated blood to the rest of the body through the aorta.

Maintaining a healthy circulatory system is crucial for optimal chicken health. Proper nutrition, including a balanced diet rich in essential vitamins and minerals, is vital for supporting the production of healthy blood cells. Adequate hydration is also necessary to ensure blood volume remains at optimal levels. Regular exercise and minimizing stress factors can contribute to maintaining a healthy heart and circulatory system in chickens.

Understanding the processes of breathing and circulating blood is essential for maintaining optimal chicken health. Proper ventilation and respiratory hygiene help prevent respiratory ailments, while a healthy circulatory system ensures the delivery of oxygen and nutrients throughout a chicken's body. By prioritizing these aspects and implementing appropriate measures, chicken owners can safeguard the well-being of their feathered friends and promote a thriving poultry flock. Remember, a healthy chicken is a happy chicken!

Eating and digestion

In the realm of poultry health, it is imperative to understand the intricacies of eating and digestion in chickens. A balanced diet and efficient digestive system are key factors that contribute to the overall well-being of these feathered creatures. This article delves into the fascinating world of eating and digestion in chickens, shedding light on their dietary requirements, digestive processes, and essential tips for promoting optimal health.

1. **The Importance of a Balanced Diet:** A balanced diet is crucial for the growth, development, and productivity of chickens. It provides the necessary nutrients, vitamins, and minerals to maintain their health and vitality. The primary components of a chicken's diet include grains, protein sources, minerals, vitamins, and water. Proper nutrition not only helps chickens achieve their full growth potential but also enhances their immune system, bone strength, egg production, and meat quality.

Digestive System of Chickens:

The digestive system of chickens is uniquely adapted to handle their dietary needs. The journey of food begins as they peck and swallow it, moving it into the crop—a pouch-like organ in the throat. From the crop, the food enters the proventriculus, where gastric juices start breaking it down. Next, it passes through the gizzard, a muscular organ lined with tough tissues and small stones, which helps grind the food into smaller particles. The food then reaches the small intestine, where enzymes break down proteins, carbohydrates, and fats for absorption. Finally, the undigested residue enters the large intestine, where water absorption takes place, and waste is formed.

Promoting Healthy Digestion:

1. **High-Quality Feed:** Provide chickens with a well-balanced, commercially formulated feed that meets their specific nutritional requirements. This ensures they receive the essential nutrients in the right proportions.
2. **Access to Clean Water:** Fresh and clean water should be available at all times. Hydration is crucial for digestion, nutrient absorption, and overall health. Ensure water sources are regularly cleaned to prevent bacterial contamination.
3. **Grit and Supplements:** Chickens require grit (small stones or gravel) to aid in the grinding process in their gizzard. Additionally, certain supplements such as calcium, vitamin D, and probiotics can be beneficial for their digestive health. Consult a poultry nutritionist or veterinarian for specific recommendations.
4. **Avoid Overfeeding:** Overfeeding can lead to obesity, digestive problems, and reduced egg production. Feed chickens according to their age, breed, and recommended portion sizes.
5. **Provide Adequate Fiber:** Including some fibrous materials like hay or leafy greens in their diet can help stimulate their digestive system and prevent issues like impacted crops.
6. **Monitor Health:** Regularly observe the birds for any signs of digestive issues such as diarrhea, bloating, or reduced appetite. Consult a veterinarian if any concerns arise.

Understanding the importance of eating and digestion is vital for maintaining the health and well-being of chickens. A well-balanced diet, a properly functioning digestive system, and good husbandry practices contribute to optimal growth, productivity, and disease resistance in these remarkable birds. By following the guidelines outlined in the Chicken Health Bible, poultry owners can ensure that their chickens thrive and lead healthy lives. Remember, a healthy digestive system paves the way for healthy chickens!

The skeletal system

In the realm of chicken health, it is essential to understand the significance of the skeletal system. The skeletal system forms the framework upon which a chicken's body is built, providing support, protection, and mobility. A strong and healthy skeletal system is vital for chickens to lead active and productive lives. This article delves into the importance of the skeletal system within the context of chicken health, offering insights into its structure, function, and strategies for maintaining skeletal well-being.

Structure and Composition:

The skeletal system of a chicken consists of bones, joints, cartilage, and connective tissues. The bones provide the structural framework and are composed primarily of calcium, phosphorus, and collagen. The framework consists of two main components: the axial skeleton, which includes the skull, backbone, and ribs, and the appendicular skeleton, consisting of the wings, legs, and pelvic bones.

Functions of the Skeletal System:

1. **Support and Protection:** The skeletal system serves as a sturdy framework that supports the chicken's body weight and internal organs. It provides protection to vital organs such as the heart, lungs, and brain, safeguarding them from potential injuries.
2. **Mobility:** The bones and joints of the skeletal system work in unison to facilitate movement. The articulation of bones at joints allows chickens to walk, run, flap their wings, and engage in various physical activities.
3. **Calcium Homeostasis:** Chickens require a steady supply of calcium for egg production and overall health. The skeletal system acts as a reservoir for calcium, allowing the body to maintain adequate levels of this mineral. When calcium intake from the diet is insufficient, the body can mobilize calcium from the bones to meet the needs of other vital functions.

Common Skeletal Issues in Chickens:

1. **Osteoporosis:** Calcium deficiency can lead to weakened bones, resulting in osteoporosis. Inadequate calcium levels in the diet or poor absorption can contribute to this condition. Chickens affected by osteoporosis are prone to bone fractures, lameness, and decreased eggshell quality.
2. **Leg Disorders:** Leg-related problems, such as slipped tendons, twisted legs, and splayed legs, can occur due to genetic factors, nutritional imbalances, or poor environmental conditions. These issues affect the chicken's ability to walk and lead to discomfort and reduced mobility.
3. **Bone Deformities:** Nutritional deficiencies, especially in calcium, phosphorus, and vitamin D3, can lead to skeletal deformities in chickens. Conditions like rickets, characterized by weak and deformed bones, can impair growth and overall well-being.

Maintaining Skeletal Health:

1. **Balanced Nutrition**: A well-rounded diet is crucial for maintaining skeletal health in chickens. Providing a balanced feed that includes adequate levels of calcium, phosphorus, and essential vitamins and minerals is essential. Consider offering calcium supplements, especially during periods of increased egg production.
2. **Environmental Considerations:** Providing a clean and spacious environment for chickens is important to minimize the risk of injuries. Ensure that the coop has suitable flooring and bedding materials to reduce strain on the legs and joints.
3. **Regular Exercise:** Allowing chickens ample space for exercise and free-ranging promotes natural movement, which aids in maintaining strong bones and joints. Encourage natural foraging behaviors to engage their muscles and promote mobility.
4. **Veterinary Care:** Regular check-ups by a poultry veterinarian can help identify and address skeletal issues at an early stage. They can provide advice on specific nutritional

requirements and recommend appropriate supplements if needed.

The skeletal system plays a pivotal role in the overall health and well-being of chickens. A robust and well-maintained skeletal system ensures mobility, supports organ function, and protects against injuries. By prioritizing balanced nutrition, providing suitable environmental conditions, and promoting regular exercise, chicken owners can help ensure optimal skeletal health for their flock.

The Chicken and then the Egg

The chicken and the egg have long been the subject of a thought-provoking riddle: Which came first, the chicken or the egg? While the question may seem perplexing, understanding the life cycle of a chicken sheds light on this age-old mystery. In this article, we will delve into the growth and development of chickens, from reaching sexual maturity to the intricate process of egg production. Furthermore, we will explore what happens within the egg and the crucial early weeks of a chick's life.

Growth and Development:

Chickens, like most birds, go through a fascinating process of growth and development. They start their lives as eggs and progress through various stages before hatching into adorable chicks. The entire journey begins when a mature hen lays an egg.

Reaching Sexual Maturity:

For a chicken to lay eggs, it must first reach sexual maturity. Typically, hens reach this stage around five to six months of age, although it can vary depending on the breed. At this point, the hen's reproductive system becomes fully functional, and it starts producing eggs. Roosters, on the other hand, mature earlier and develop their distinct crowing and mating behaviors.

Making Eggs (and Chicks, maybe):

Once a hen reaches sexual maturity, it can lay eggs regularly. The process of egg formation occurs within the hen's body. The hen's reproductive system includes ovaries, where the eggs develop. Each ovary contains thousands of tiny ova (egg cells), and one ovum matures into an egg during each reproductive cycle.

Knowing what goes on in the egg:

Inside the hen's body, a yolk forms and starts its journey through the oviduct. The yolk gathers nutrients along the way and eventually enters the shell gland, where the eggshell is formed. The shell gland secretes calcium carbonate, providing strength and protection to the developing chick within the egg. The egg is then laid, and if fertilized by a rooster, it has the potential to develop into a chick.

A Chick's First Few Weeks:

When a fertilized egg is incubated under appropriate conditions, it undergoes a mesmerizing transformation. The chick develops within the egg, drawing nutrients from the yolk and breathing through the porous eggshell. After approximately 21 days of incubation, the chick begins to peck its way out of the shell using a specialized structure called an egg tooth.

Once hatched, the chick enters the world with downy feathers and a strong instinct to explore its surroundings. It relies on the nutrition stored in the yolk sac for sustenance during its first days. The chick's early weeks are crucial for proper growth and development, and it requires a warm and safe environment, proper nutrition, and protection from predators.

The chicken and the egg puzzle capture our curiosity and imagination, but understanding the life cycle of chickens unravels the mystery. From reaching sexual maturity to egg production, and the incredible development of chicks within the egg, the journey of a chicken is truly awe-inspiring. By learning about their growth and development, we can better appreciate the vital role chickens play in providing us with eggs and nourishment. Whether you prefer scrambled, fried, or boiled, the chicken's remarkable life cycle is an essential part of the story behind our breakfast table.

Chapter 7

Signs Of Chicken Illness

Welcome to Chapter 7 of the Chicken Health Bible, where we delve into the crucial topic of recognizing signs of chicken illness. As poultry keepers, it is our responsibility to ensure the well-being of our feathered friends, and being able to identify symptoms of illness is an essential skill in maintaining a healthy flock.

Chickens, like any living creatures, are susceptible to various diseases and health issues. Whether you are a seasoned chicken keeper or just starting your journey, being familiar with the signs of illness is vital for early detection and prompt intervention, which can significantly improve the chances of recovery.

In this chapter, we will explore the different indicators that can help you identify if a chicken is unwell. We'll cover both general signs of illness and specific symptoms related to various common chicken diseases. By understanding these signals, you will be better equipped to take appropriate action and seek necessary veterinary assistance when needed.

Some of the key topics we will discuss include changes in behavior, such as lethargy or unusual aggression, as well as physical signs like abnormal feather appearance, weight loss, respiratory distress, and changes in droppings. We will also examine specific symptoms associated with prevalent chicken diseases, such as avian influenza, coccidiosis, Marek's disease, and others.

It is important to note that while this chapter will provide valuable insights into recognizing signs of chicken illness, it should not replace professional veterinary advice. If you suspect that your chicken is unwell, consulting with an avian veterinarian is always recommended to ensure accurate diagnosis and appropriate treatment.

By becoming familiar with the signs of chicken illness, you will be able to take proactive steps to protect the health and well-being of your flock. Early detection and timely intervention can not only save individual birds but also prevent the spread of contagious diseases among the entire flock.

So, let's embark on this important journey of understanding the signs of chicken illness. By the end of this chapter, you will have a solid foundation for recognizing when your chickens need your attention and care. Together, let's ensure a healthier and happier flock!

Recognizing the General Signs of Illness

Welcome to the world of chicken health! If you're a poultry owner or simply fascinated by these feathered creatures, it's crucial to have a basic understanding of how to recognize the general signs of illness in your chickens. By being observant and proactive, you can ensure the well-being of your flock and address any potential health concerns promptly.

The "Chicken Health Bible" is an invaluable resource that will guide you through various aspects of chicken health, including disease recognition, prevention, and treatment. In this introductory content, we will focus on recognizing the general signs of illness in chickens, providing you with a foundation for understanding and caring for your feathered friends.

Chickens, like any living beings, can fall ill due to a variety of reasons, including viral, bacterial, and fungal infections, as well as parasites and nutritional deficiencies. It's important to note that different illnesses may present different symptoms, but there are some common signs that may indicate your chicken is unwell.

Changes in behavior:

Keep an eye out for any abnormal behavior in your chickens. This could include lethargy, a decrease in appetite, increased aggression, or a general withdrawal from the flock. Chickens are social animals, so any sudden change in their behavior may indicate an underlying health issue.

Abnormal droppings:

Pay attention to the color, consistency, and frequency of your chickens' droppings. Healthy droppings should be firm, with a dark brown or greenish color. Watery, bloody, or discolored droppings can indicate intestinal issues, infections, or parasites.

Respiratory issues:

Observe your chickens' breathing patterns. If you notice any wheezing, coughing, sneezing, or gasping for breath, it could be a sign of respiratory problems such as infectious bronchitis or Newcastle disease.

Changes in appearance:

A healthy chicken should have bright eyes, clean feathers, and a well-groomed appearance. Look for any signs of disheveled feathers, ruffled appearance, or unusual growths on the skin. These could be indicators of external parasites or skin infections.

Changes in egg production:

If your hens suddenly stop laying eggs or there's a significant decrease in egg production, it may signal an underlying health issue. Reproductive problems, nutritional imbalances, or infections can all impact egg-laying abilities.

Remember, this introductory content is just the tip of the iceberg when it comes to recognizing signs of illness in chickens. The "Chicken Health Bible" will provide you with comprehensive knowledge and guidance to help you become a knowledgeable and proactive poultry owner.

By regularly observing your chickens and being aware of these general signs of illness, you can catch potential health problems early on and seek appropriate veterinary care or implement necessary preventive measures. Your commitment to the well-being of your flock will contribute to their overall health and happiness. So, let's dive into the world of chicken health and start on this rewarding journey together!

The Physical Examination

In the world of poultry farming, maintaining the health and well-being of chickens is of paramount importance. A comprehensive understanding of chicken health and the ability to detect potential issues early on is essential for successful poultry management. The physical examination plays a vital role in assessing the overall health of chickens, identifying potential problems, and ensuring timely intervention. In this article, we will explore the significance of the physical examination within the context of the Chicken Health Bible.

Importance of Physical Examination:

1. **Early Detection of Health Issues:** Regular physical examinations enable poultry farmers to identify potential health problems in chickens at an early stage. By observing their appearance, behavior, and physical condition, farmers can spot signs of illness, injury, or disease. Early detection allows for prompt treatment, minimizing the risk of spreading diseases within the flock and reducing the chances of severe complications.
2. **Preventive Measures:** Physical examinations are not only about identifying existing health problems but also about implementing preventive measures. By closely examining chickens, farmers can identify risk factors and take proactive steps to prevent diseases. This may include maintaining proper biosecurity measures, optimizing nutrition, and ensuring appropriate housing conditions.

Components of a Physical Examination:

1. **General Observation:** The examination begins with a visual assessment of the chickens' overall appearance. This includes checking their body posture, feather condition, and behavior. Abnormalities such as lethargy, abnormal posture, feather loss, or disheveled feathers may indicate underlying health issues.

2. **Vital Signs:** Similar to humans, monitoring vital signs is crucial in assessing chicken health. This involves evaluating respiratory rate, heart rate, and body temperature. Deviations from normal values would indicate respiratory infections, cardiovascular problems, or fever.
3. **Skin and Feather Examination:** The condition of the skin and feathers provides important clues about the chickens' overall health. Any signs of parasites, such as lice or mites, should be noted. Skin lesions, scabs, or abnormal feather loss might indicate infectious or dermatological conditions.
4. **Eye, Ear, and Beak Inspection:** Examination of the eyes, ears, and beak helps identify potential issues. Watery or discolored eyes may indicate respiratory infections or conjunctivitis. Swelling or discharge from the ears could be a sign of ear infections. The beak should be examined for deformities or signs of injury.
5. **Abdominal Palpation:** Gentle palpation of the abdomen allows farmers to check for abnormalities such as abdominal distention, tumors, or egg-binding in hens. Any signs of pain or discomfort during palpation require further investigation.

The physical examination is a fundamental tool in the Chicken Health Bible, aiding poultry farmers in maintaining optimal chicken health. By regularly observing and assessing chickens' appearance, behavior, and physical condition, farmers can identify potential health issues at an early stage, implement preventive measures, and ensure prompt treatment when needed. Through diligent physical examinations, poultry farmers can contribute to the overall well-being and productivity of their flocks, promoting a sustainable and successful poultry farming enterprise.

Catching and holding the sick chicken

Keeping a flock of healthy chickens is a rewarding experience, but occasionally, chickens may fall ill. As a responsible chicken owner, it's crucial to be prepared to handle sick birds with care and attention. Catching and holding a sick chicken correctly can minimize stress for both the bird and you while ensuring the best chances for a successful recovery. This guide will provide you with essential tips on catching and holding a sick chicken, emphasizing their comfort, safety, and well-being.

Observe and Assess:

Before attempting to catch a sick chicken, carefully observe their behavior and physical condition. Look for any signs of illness such as lethargy, loss of appetite, abnormal droppings, respiratory distress, or changes in behavior. This information will help you determine the severity of the illness and whether veterinary intervention is necessary.

Gather Supplies:

Before handling a sick chicken, gather the necessary supplies. These may include gloves, a towel, a small box or carrier, and any medications or treatments prescribed by a veterinarian. Having these items readily available will make the process smoother and minimize stress for the bird.

Approach Calmly:

Approach the sick chicken slowly and calmly. Abrupt movements or loud noises can startle the bird, causing additional stress and making it more difficult to catch. Speak softly and move with gentle, deliberate motions to avoid alarming the chicken.

Secure the Chicken:

To catch a sick chicken, it's best to approach from behind. With one hand, gently grasp the bird's body around the wings, being careful not to squeeze too tightly. Use your other hand to support the bird's legs, holding them securely but not forcefully. Lift the chicken slowly and smoothly, keeping its body close to your chest.

Provide Support and Comfort:

While holding the sick chicken, maintain a secure grip while being mindful of its comfort. Chickens are fragile creatures, and they may be weakened by illness. Use a soft towel or cloth to provide a stable and comfortable surface for the bird to rest on while you examine or administer any necessary treatments.

Minimize Stress:

Minimizing stress is crucial for a sick chicken's recovery. Keep handling time to a minimum and handle the bird gently. Avoid sudden movements, loud noises, or exposing the chicken to extreme temperatures during the process. If you need to transport the bird, ensure the carrier or box is well-ventilated, secure, and provides sufficient space for the chicken to stand or lie down comfortably.

Seek Veterinary Assistance:

While you can provide basic care for a sick chicken, it's essential to consult a veterinarian for a proper diagnosis and treatment plan. Veterinarians can provide guidance specific to the bird's condition and may prescribe medications or recommend supportive care measures to aid in the recovery process. Catching and holding a sick chicken requires patience, gentleness, and a focus on the bird's well-being. By approaching the process calmly, securing the chicken properly, and minimizing stress, you can ensure that both you and the bird remain safe and comfortable. Remember to consult with a veterinarian for professional guidance to provide the best possible care for your sick chicken. With proper handling and veterinary care, the chances of a successful recovery increase, allowing your flock to thrive once again.

Examining the head

The health and well-being of chickens are essential for backyard poultry keepers and commercial farmers alike. When it comes to assessing the overall health of a chicken, examining the head is a crucial aspect. By observing the head, poultry owners can detect potential issues early on and take appropriate measures to ensure the birds' welfare. In this article, we will delve into the significance of examining the head of chickens and provide valuable insights into common head-related health conditions.

The Head as a Window to Overall Health:

The head of a chicken serves as a gateway to understanding its overall well-being. By paying attention to specific areas of the head, poultry owners can gain valuable information about the chicken's physical condition, behavior, and potential health concerns. Examining the head allows for early detection of various issues that may affect a chicken's ability to eat, breathe, see, and communicate.

Key Areas of Examination:

1. **Eyes:** Clear, bright eyes are signs of a healthy chicken. Observe for any discharge, swelling, redness, or cloudiness, which may indicate eye infections, respiratory problems, or nutritional deficiencies.
2. **Beak**: The beak should be straight, symmetrical, and free from deformities. Check for any signs of cracking, lesions, or abnormal growth, which might indicate nutritional imbalances or infectious diseases.
3. **Comb and Wattles**: These fleshy, red structures on top of the chicken's head should be vibrant in color. Pale or discolored combs and wattles may suggest anemia, poor blood circulation, or heat stress.
4. **Nostrils:** Clear, open nostrils are essential for proper respiration. Look for any discharge, blockages, or signs of respiratory distress, as they could be indications of respiratory infections or respiratory parasites.
5. **Head Movements:** Observe the chicken's head movements for any abnormalities such as excessive shaking, nodding, or tilting. These behaviors may be indicative of neurological disorders or ear infections.

Common Head-Related Health Conditions:

1. **Respiratory Infections:** Infectious diseases like Mycoplasma gallisepticum or Infectious Coryza can cause symptoms like swollen sinuses, nasal discharge, and respiratory distress.
2. **Eye Infections:** Conjunctivitis, or "Pink Eye," is a common bacterial infection that causes redness, swelling, and discharge from the eyes. It can be caused by poor hygiene, dust, or bacterial contamination.
3. **Nutritional Deficiencies:** Inadequate nutrition can manifest in the head region, leading to beak abnormalities, pale combs, wattles, and dull eyes. Ensure a balanced diet with proper vitamins, minerals, and protein.
4. **Head Trauma:** Accidents or aggressive behavior from other chickens can cause head injuries, leading to swelling, bleeding, or fractures. Prompt veterinary care is essential to prevent further complications.

Prevention and Care:

1. Maintain a clean and hygienic environment for your chickens, ensuring proper ventilation and regular cleaning of coop bedding.
2. Provide a well-balanced, nutrient-rich diet to meet the chickens' nutritional needs.
3. Quarantine new birds before introducing them to the flock to prevent the spread of diseases.
4. Perform regular health checks, including head examination, to monitor any changes or abnormalities.
5. Consult a veterinarian if you notice persistent or concerning symptoms in your chickens.

Examining the head of chickens is a critical aspect of monitoring their health. By observing key areas and being attentive to any changes or abnormalities, poultry owners can detect potential health issues early on, allowing for prompt intervention and treatment. Maintaining good hygiene, providing proper nutrition, and seeking professional advice when needed will contribute to the overall well-being and vitality of your flock. Remember, a healthy head leads to a happy and thriving chicken!

Looking at skin and feathers

In the fascinating world of poultry, chickens are undoubtedly the most popular and widely-raised birds. These feathery creatures not only provide us with delicious eggs and meat but also offer companionship and entertainment. Just like any living being, chickens require proper care and attention to ensure their overall health and well-being. When it comes to assessing their health, examining their skin and feathers can provide valuable insights. In this article, we delve into the topic of looking at skin and feathers as part of the Chicken Health Bible.

The skin and feathers of a chicken serve multiple purposes, including protection, insulation, and communication. They also act as indicators of the bird's overall health and can reveal potential issues that need attention. By observing and understanding the condition of a chicken's skin and feathers, poultry owners can detect early signs of illness, manage existing conditions, and take proactive measures to maintain optimal health.

Firstly, let's explore the significance of examining a chicken's skin. A healthy chicken should have smooth and supple skin. When assessing the skin, look for any abnormalities such as redness, swelling, lesions, or scabs. These could be signs of external parasites like mites or lice, which can cause discomfort and lead to further health complications if left untreated. In addition, keep an eye out for excessive dryness or flakiness, as it may indicate poor nutrition or environmental factors that need to be addressed. A chicken's skin should be free from wounds, cuts, or any signs of infection, which could require veterinary intervention.

Moving on to feathers, they play a crucial role in a chicken's life. Feathers not only help birds maintain their body temperature but also aid in flight, mating rituals, and protection from predators. The quality and appearance of feathers can provide valuable insights into a chicken's overall health. Healthy feathers are smooth, glossy, and well-arranged. They should have a consistent color and show no signs of bald patches, discoloration, or excessive shedding.

Feather abnormalities can indicate various health issues. Feather pecking or plucking can be a behavioral problem caused by stress, boredom, or overcrowding. Feather loss may also result from external parasites, nutritional deficiencies, or underlying diseases. Additionally, matted or dirty feathers may suggest poor hygiene or infestations. It is essential to investigate and address the underlying cause of any feather irregularities to prevent further complications and ensure the bird's well-being.

Regular grooming and maintenance are vital for maintaining healthy skin and feathers in chickens. This includes providing a clean and comfortable living environment, a balanced and nutritious diet, and appropriate protection against external parasites. Regularly inspecting the skin and feathers during routine health checks can help detect any abnormalities early on, allowing for prompt intervention and treatment if necessary.

Looking at a chicken's skin and feathers is an important aspect of monitoring their health and well-being. By understanding what to observe and what signs to look for, poultry owners can ensure early detection of potential issues and take appropriate measures to maintain optimal health. Remember, a healthy chicken with vibrant feathers and smooth skin is not only a joy to behold but also a testament to responsible and caring poultry management.

Looking at wings, legs, and feet

In the vast world of backyard poultry keeping, ensuring the health and well-being of your chickens is of utmost importance. A healthy chicken is a happy chicken, and observing their wings, legs, and feet can provide valuable insights into their overall health. In this article, we will explore how these body parts can serve as indicators of your chickens' well-being and discuss common issues that may arise.

The Wings:

A chicken's wings are not only essential for their ability to fly short distances but also reveal valuable information about their health. When examining the wings, check for any signs of feather loss, damage, or excessive molting. Feather loss can be a result of external parasites such as mites or lice, which can cause discomfort and lead to other health issues if left untreated. Observe the wings for signs of redness, swelling, or lesions, which could indicate an infection or injury.

Additionally, pay attention to the wing motion when your chickens are walking or stretching their wings. Restricted wing movement or a noticeable limp may suggest a muscular or skeletal issue that requires attention. Regular wing clipping is also recommended to prevent injury or escape attempts, as well as to maintain balance during flight.

The Legs:

Chicken legs play a crucial role in supporting their body weight and facilitating movement. Therefore, observing their legs can help identify potential health concerns. Start by examining the scales on their legs and feet. Healthy scales are smooth and well-defined, while rough or raised scales may indicate an underlying issue.

Swelling, redness, or heat in the legs can be signs of inflammation or infection, such as bumblefoot. Bumblefoot is a common condition characterized by a bacterial infection in the footpad, often caused by rough surfaces or injury. Early detection and treatment are essential to prevent the infection from spreading and causing further complications.

It's also important to pay attention to the leg and foot posture of your chickens. A chicken standing or walking with a hunched posture, favoring one leg, or struggling to put weight on a leg may be experiencing pain or injury. Such conditions could result from fractures, sprains, or joint problems and should be addressed promptly to alleviate discomfort and prevent long-term damage.

The Feet:

Chicken feet are intricate structures that aid in balance, perching, and foraging. Healthy feet are characterized by well-trimmed nails and clean, unswollen footpads. Overgrown nails can cause discomfort and may lead to issues with walking or perching. Regular nail trimming is crucial to prevent these problems and maintain good foot health.

Inspect the footpads for any signs of injury, swelling, or ulceration. Footpad lesions can be caused by standing on abrasive or dirty surfaces or by a condition known as "scald" due to prolonged exposure to damp litter. Keeping their environment clean and dry is vital to prevent foot pad issues.

Monitoring the wings, legs, and feet of your chickens is a crucial aspect of maintaining their overall health and well-being. By paying attention to any changes or abnormalities in these body parts, you can identify potential health issues early on and provide timely care. Regular observation, proper hygiene, and preventive measures, such as wing clipping and nail trimming, can help keep your chickens in top condition. Remember, a healthy chicken is a happy chicken, and a happy chicken rewards you with delicious eggs and a lively presence in your backyard.

Checking the abdomen and vent

As a poultry keeper, it is essential to regularly check the health and well-being of your chickens. One crucial aspect of this is examining their abdomen and vent. By paying attention to these areas, you can detect any signs of discomfort or disease early on, ensuring prompt intervention and maintaining the overall health of your flock. In this article, we will explore the significance of checking the abdomen and vent of your chickens and provide you with a comprehensive guide to doing so effectively.

Importance of Abdomen and Vent Examination:

The abdomen and vent are areas that can offer valuable insights into a chicken's health. By examining these regions regularly, you can detect potential issues such as infections, injuries, or blockages. Here are some reasons why checking the abdomen and vent is crucial:

1. **Disease Prevention:** Early detection of diseases or abnormalities in the abdomen and vent can prevent the spread of infections and potentially save the lives of your chickens.
2. **Comfort and Well-being:** Issues in the abdomen or vent area, such as egg binding or prolapse, can cause significant discomfort to your chickens. By identifying and addressing these problems promptly, you can alleviate their suffering and promote their well-being.
3. **Reproductive Health:** The vent is the opening through which hens lay eggs. Monitoring this area helps ensure the reproductive health of your flock, ensuring the smooth passage of eggs and preventing complications.

How to Check the Abdomen and Vent:

1. **Prepare a suitable space:** Find a clean and well-lit area where you can comfortably examine your chicken. Ensure that you have a good light source and any necessary tools, such as gloves, clean towels, and lubricant, within reach.
2. **Gentle Restraint:** Approach the chicken calmly and securely restrain it, gently holding its wings against its body to prevent flapping. This will keep the chicken calm and allow for a more accurate examination.
3. **Abdomen Examination:** Carefully lift the chicken's feathers around the vent area and observe the abdomen. Look for any swelling, lumps, or abnormalities. Palpate the abdomen gently, feeling for any unusual masses or fluid build-up.
4. **Vent Examination:** With clean hands or gloved fingers, examine the vent. Check for any signs of irritation, inflammation, or discharge. In laying hens, ensure the vent is clean and free from any stuck eggshell fragments or abnormal protrusions.
5. **Egg Binding and Prolapse:** If you suspect egg binding (difficulty laying eggs) or prolapse (when internal organs protrude from the vent), it is crucial to seek veterinary assistance immediately. These conditions can be life-threatening and require professional intervention.
6. **Regular Hygiene:** After examination, clean the vent area if necessary. Use warm water and a mild, poultry-safe cleanser to gently wash away any debris or buildup. Ensure the area is thoroughly dried before returning the chicken to its coop.

Checking the abdomen and vent of your chickens is an essential part of maintaining their health and preventing potential complications. By regularly examining these areas, you can identify and address any issues promptly, ensuring the well-being of your flock. Remember, if you notice any abnormalities or are unsure about what you observe, consult with a veterinarian who specializes in poultry health. With consistent care and attention, you can help your chickens lead happy and healthy lives.

Chapter 8

Common Illnesses In Adult Chickens

Maintaining the health of your chickens is crucial for their overall well-being and productivity. One common issue that chicken owners may encounter is respiratory illness. Chicken respiratory illnesses, often referred to as chicken head colds, can affect the respiratory system of your flock, leading to symptoms such as coughing, sneezing, nasal discharge, and reduced egg production. In this article, we will discuss how to diagnose chicken respiratory illness and provide supportive care to help your chickens recover.

Diagnosing Chicken Respiratory Illness:

1. **Observe Symptoms:** The first step in diagnosing chicken respiratory illness is to closely observe your flock for any signs of respiratory distress. Look for symptoms such as coughing, sneezing, wheezing, nasal discharge, labored breathing, or a rattling sound when breathing.
2. **Examine Affected Birds:** Once you notice these symptoms, it is important to separate the affected chickens from the rest of the flock to prevent the spread of infection. Carefully examine the affected birds for any visible signs of illness, such as swollen eyes, mucus in the beak, or inflamed sinuses.
3. **Seek Veterinary Assistance:** If the symptoms persist or worsen, it is recommended to consult a veterinarian experienced in poultry care. They can conduct further diagnostic tests, such as swabs, blood tests, or cultures, to identify the specific respiratory illness affecting your flock.

Giving Supportive Care for Chicken Respiratory Illness:

1. **Isolate and Quarantine:** As soon as you notice any respiratory symptoms in your chickens, isolate the affected birds in a separate, well-ventilated area. Quarantining the sick birds prevents the spread of the illness to healthy members of the flock.
2. **Improve Ventilation:** Proper ventilation is crucial for reducing the spread of respiratory infections and aiding the recovery of infected birds. Ensure that the chicken coop or housing area has adequate airflow while avoiding drafts that may exacerbate the illness. Ventilation helps maintain a clean and dry environment, preventing the buildup of harmful bacteria.
3. **Provide Clean Water and Nutritious Feed:** To support the immune system of your chickens, ensure they have access to clean, fresh water at all times. Offer a balanced diet with high-quality feed that contains essential nutrients and vitamins to boost their overall health and recovery.
4. **Promote Hygiene:** Maintain good hygiene practices by regularly cleaning the coop, removing damp bedding, and disinfecting the area. Regularly sanitize feeders and waterers to prevent bacterial growth and contamination.
5. **Offer Warmth:** During illness, chickens may benefit from additional warmth. Provide a heat source, such as a heat lamp, in the isolation area to keep the birds comfortable and promote healing.
6. **Administer Medications (if prescribed):** Depending on the specific diagnosis, your veterinarian may prescribe antibiotics or other medications to treat the respiratory illness. Administer the medications as directed, following the proper dosage and duration.

Diagnosing and providing supportive care for chicken respiratory illness is essential for the health and recovery of your flock. By observing symptoms, seeking veterinary assistance, and implementing proper supportive care measures such as isolation, ventilation, nutrition, hygiene, and warmth, you can help your chickens overcome respiratory illnesses and maintain a healthy and productive flock. Remember, prevention is key, so always strive to maintain a clean and hygienic environment to minimize the risk of respiratory infections in your chickens.

Diarrhea in Adult Chickens

Diarrhea is a common health issue in adult chickens that can significantly impact their well-being and productivity. Timely diagnosis and appropriate supportive care are essential to manage this condition effectively. In this article, we will explore the process of diagnosing diarrhea in adult chickens and discuss the necessary measures for providing supportive care.

Diagnosing Diarrhea in Adult Chickens:

1. **Visual Observation:** The initial step in diagnosing diarrhea involves visually inspecting the chicken's droppings. Normal droppings in adult chickens consist of a dark, firm fecal component (called the feces) and a white, semi-solid component (urates). Diarrhea is indicated by the presence of loose, watery, or excessively liquid feces.

2. **Consistency and Color:** Assessing the consistency and color of the droppings is crucial. Diarrhea can manifest as extremely watery or foamy droppings, and the color may range from yellow to green or even contain blood.
3. **Odor and Frequency:** Pay attention to any abnormal odor associated with the droppings, such as a foul smell. Additionally, note the frequency of defecation, as an increase in the number of bowel movements can be indicative of diarrhea.
4. **Environmental Factors:** Consider the overall environment in which the chickens are kept. Poor sanitation, overcrowding, contaminated water, or improper diet can contribute to the development of diarrhea. Identifying and addressing these factors is important for managing the condition effectively.

Giving Supportive Care for Adult Chickens with Diarrhea:

1. **Isolation:** If a chicken is diagnosed with diarrhea, isolate it from the rest of the flock to prevent the spread of any potential infections. This will also allow you to closely monitor its condition and ensure it receives proper care.
2. **Hydration:** Diarrhea can cause dehydration, so it is crucial to provide clean and fresh water at all times. Consider adding electrolytes or vitamins to the water to replenish any lost nutrients. Offer small amounts of water frequently to encourage hydration.
3. **Nutritional Management:** Adjust the chicken's diet to promote healing and recovery. Provide easily digestible, low-fiber foods such as cooked rice, plain boiled chicken, or commercial chicken feeds specifically designed for sick birds. Avoid feeding fruits, vegetables, or other high-fiber foods during this time.
4. **Medication and Probiotics:** Consult with a veterinarian to determine if medication or probiotics are necessary for the chicken's condition. Antibiotics may be prescribed if a bacterial infection is suspected, while probiotics can help restore a healthy balance of gut bacteria.
5. **Clean Environment:** Ensure the chicken's living area is clean and free from fecal contamination. Regularly remove soiled bedding and disinfect the coop to minimize the risk of reinfection or the spread of pathogens.
6. **Veterinary Consultation:** If the chicken's diarrhea persists or worsens despite supportive care, seek veterinary assistance. A professional opinion can help identify underlying causes or recommend additional treatment options.

Diagnosing and managing diarrhea in adult chickens requires careful observation and appropriate supportive care. By closely monitoring the droppings, addressing environmental factors, providing isolation, maintaining hydration, adjusting the diet, and seeking veterinary guidance when needed, you can effectively support the affected chickens and aid in their recovery. Remember, prevention is key, so maintaining good hygiene practices and providing a balanced diet are crucial for minimizing the occurrence of diarrhea in your flock.

Egg-Binding and Vent Prolapse

Keeping a flock of chickens requires careful attention to their health and well-being. While chickens are generally resilient creatures, they can sometimes experience health issues such as egg-binding and vent prolapse. These conditions can be distressing for both the chicken and its caretaker, but with proper knowledge and prompt action, they can often be successfully treated. In this article, we will explore how to identify these conditions, provide appropriate treatment, and offer general care guidelines for chickens facing egg-binding and vent prolapse.

Identifying Egg-Binding:

Egg-binding, also known as egg dystocia, occurs when a hen is unable to pass an egg. This condition can be caused by several factors, including genetics, poor nutrition, obesity, inadequate calcium levels, or abnormalities in the reproductive system. Here are some signs to look out for when identifying egg-binding in chickens:

1. **Lethargy and weakness:** Affected chickens may exhibit a lack of energy and appear weak or uninterested in their surroundings.
2. **Distended abdomen:** An enlarged or swollen abdomen is a common symptom of egg-binding.
3. **Straining and vocalization**: Chickens experiencing egg-binding may strain while attempting to pass the egg, often accompanied by vocalization or distress sounds.
4. **Decreased appetite and water intake:** Egg-bound hens may show a reduced interest in food and water.
5. **Prolonged time spent in the nest box:** If a chicken spends an unusually long time in the nest box without laying an egg, it may indicate egg-binding.

Identifying Vent Prolapse:

Vent prolapse, also known as cloacal prolapse, is a condition in which the lower part of the chicken's digestive and reproductive tract protrudes through the vent. This can occur due to excessive straining, reproductive abnormalities, egg-binding, or trauma. Here are some signs to look out for when identifying vent prolapse in chickens:

1. **Visible tissue protrusion:** A reddish or pinkish bulge of tissue outside the vent area is a clear indicator of vent prolapse.
2. **Swelling and irritation:** The prolapsed tissue may appear swollen, inflamed, or irritated.
3. **Discomfort and distress:** Affected chickens may exhibit signs of discomfort, such as excessive preening, straining, or vocalization.
4. **Decreased egg production:** Vent prolapse can cause a decrease in egg-laying or even complete cessation of egg production.

Treatment and Care:

When dealing with egg-binding or vent prolapse, it is essential to take immediate action to alleviate the chicken's distress and prevent further complications. Here are some treatment and care guidelines:

1. **Isolate and provide a quiet environment:** Remove the affected chicken from the flock and place it in a separate, quiet space to reduce stress levels.
2. **Warm baths:** Soaking the chicken's lower abdomen in warm water for about 15-20 minutes, a few times a day, can help relax the muscles and potentially facilitate egg-laying.
3. **Lubrication:** Gently apply a lubricant, such as petroleum jelly or vegetable oil, to the vent area to ease the passage of the egg or reduce friction in the case of vent prolapse.
4. **Veterinary assistance**: If the chicken fails to pass the egg or if the vent prolapse is severe, consult a veterinarian for further examination and potential intervention.
5. **Calcium supplementation:** Ensure the chicken's diet is rich in calcium to support eggshell formation and prevent future egg-binding incidents.
6. **Preventive measures:** Maintain a balanced diet for your flock, provide adequate exercise opportunities, and regularly inspect nesting boxes and perches for any sharp edges or irregularities that could cause injury.

Egg-binding and vent prolapse can pose significant health risks to chickens. By promptly recognizing the signs and implementing appropriate treatment and care, chicken keepers can improve the chances of a successful outcome. However, it is important to remember that prevention is key, so maintaining a balanced diet, monitoring the health of your flock, and providing appropriate living conditions are crucial aspects of keeping chickens healthy and happy. Remember, if you are unsure or concerned about your chicken's condition, consulting a veterinarian with avian expertise is always recommended.

Egg Quality Issues

Eggs are an essential part of our daily diet, providing us with valuable nutrients and proteins. However, sometimes we may encounter egg quality issues that can affect their appearance, taste, and overall freshness. In this article, we will explore the common causes of egg quality issues and provide tips on handling odd-shaped eggs with care. This information is sourced from the "Chicken Health Bible," a comprehensive guide to maintaining the health and well-being of chickens.

Finding the Cause of Egg Quality Issues:

When it comes to egg quality issues, it's crucial to identify the underlying causes. Understanding these factors will help you take appropriate steps to prevent or address them. Here are some common issues and their potential causes:

1. **Thin or Weak Shells:** If you notice that your eggs have thin or weak shells, it may be due to nutritional deficiencies in the hens' diet. Specifically, a lack of calcium can lead to weakened shells. Ensure that your hens have access to a balanced diet that includes calcium-rich foods such as oyster shells or crushed eggshells.
2. **Oddly Shaped Eggs:** Sometimes, you may come across eggs that have unusual shapes,

such as elongated, round, or even shell-less eggs. These abnormalities can occur due to various reasons, including stress, age, genetics, or poor nutrition. Observe your flock and try to identify any stressors or dietary imbalances that may be causing these irregularities.

Handling Odd-Shaped Eggs with Care:

When you encounter odd-shaped eggs, it's essential to handle them with care to minimize any potential risks. Here are some tips to consider:

1. **Collect and Inspect Regularly:** Regularly collect eggs from the nesting boxes to ensure they don't accumulate, become dirty, or crack. Inspect each egg carefully, and if you come across any odd-shaped ones, set them aside for separate use or disposal.
2. **Wash Properly:** If an odd-shaped egg is dirty, gently clean it using warm water. Avoid using any soaps or detergents as they can remove the egg's protective cuticle, making it more susceptible to bacterial contamination.
3. **Store Separately:** If the odd-shaped egg appears intact, you can still use it for personal consumption. However, it's advisable to store it separately from the regular-shaped eggs. This separation will prevent any potential contamination from affecting the rest of the batch.
4. **Cook Thoroughly:** When using odd-shaped eggs for cooking or baking, ensure they are cooked thoroughly. Proper cooking eliminates any potential bacteria that might be present. Avoid using raw or undercooked eggs, especially in dishes like mayonnaise or meringue, which are not heated to high temperatures.

Maintaining good egg quality is essential for both consumers and poultry owners. By understanding the causes of egg quality issues and handling odd-shaped eggs with care, you can ensure a better egg-eating experience. The "Chicken Health Bible" serves as a valuable resource in providing comprehensive information on chicken health and well-being, helping you raise healthy and productive flocks. Remember to always prioritize the health and welfare of your chickens to ensure the production of high-quality eggs.

Poor Sight and Sore Eyes

Maintaining good eye health in chickens is crucial for their overall well-being. Poor sight and sore eyes can significantly impact a chicken's quality of life, affecting their ability to forage, navigate their surroundings, and interact with their flock. In this article, we will explore potential eye problems that chickens may face and discuss effective treatments to ensure their optimal eye health.

Potential Eye Problems in Chickens:

1. **Conjunctivitis:** Also known as "pink eye," conjunctivitis is a common eye condition in chickens. It is characterized by inflammation of the conjunctiva, the thin membrane that covers the inner surface of the eyelids and the white part of the eye. Conjunctivitis can be caused by bacterial or viral infections, environmental irritants, or injuries.
2. **Corneal Ulcers:** Corneal ulcers refer to the damage or erosion of the outermost layer of the

eye, the cornea. These ulcers can result from scratches caused by sharp objects or dust particles, or as a secondary infection from untreated conjunctivitis. Corneal ulcers are painful and can lead to decreased vision if left untreated.
3. **Eye Worms:** Parasitic eye worms, such as Oxyspirura mansoni, can infect chickens, causing severe discomfort and potentially leading to blindness. These worms typically reside in the eye's conjunctiva and can be transmitted through contact with intermediate hosts, such as insects.

Treatments for Eye Issues in Chickens:

1. **Veterinary Examination**: When a chicken shows signs of poor sight or sore eyes, it is essential to seek veterinary assistance. A professional examination will help determine the underlying cause of the problem and guide the appropriate treatment plan.
2. **Medication:** Depending on the diagnosis, veterinarians may prescribe ointments, eye drops, or oral medications to treat bacterial or viral infections. Antibiotics can help control bacterial conjunctivitis, while antiviral medications may be necessary for viral infections.
3. **Cleaning and Irrigation:** In cases of eye irritation or foreign objects, gentle cleaning and irrigation can help alleviate discomfort. Veterinarians may recommend using sterile saline solution or specialized eye washes to flush out any debris or irritants.
4. **Protective Measures:** To prevent further damage or infection, it is important to protect chickens with eye problems from environmental factors. This includes keeping them in clean and dust-free environments, providing proper ventilation, and minimizing contact with potential sources of eye irritation.
5. **Parasite Control:** If eye worms are diagnosed, deworming medication specifically designed for poultry can be administered. Additionally, implementing measures to control intermediate hosts, such as insects, can help reduce the risk of reinfection.

Ensuring good eye health in chickens is essential for their overall well-being. By being vigilant and proactive in identifying potential eye problems, seeking veterinary assistance, and implementing appropriate treatments, chicken owners can help alleviate discomfort, preserve vision, and enhance the quality of life for their feathered friends. Regular monitoring, maintaining clean surroundings, and practicing good hygiene can go a long way in preventing eye issues in chickens.

Skin Problems and Feather Loss

Keeping chickens healthy and thriving requires vigilance and attention to their overall well-being. One common issue that chicken owners may encounter is skin problems and feather loss. These issues can arise due to various factors, such as external parasites, nutritional deficiencies, stress, or underlying health conditions. In this article, we will explore the reasons behind skin problems and feather loss in chickens and provide effective strategies to soothe these issues, ensuring the well-being of your feathered friends.

Noticing feather and skin issues: Observing changes in your chicken's feathers and skin is essential for identifying potential problems. Here are some common signs to watch out for:

1. **Feather loss:** Excessive shedding or bald patches on your chicken's body or wings could indicate a problem.
2. **Irritated or red skin:** Inflamed or reddened skin, especially in specific areas, may suggest an underlying issue.
3. **Pecking or scratching:** If your chickens are excessively pecking or scratching their feathers, it could be a sign of skin discomfort or irritation.
4. **Scaly or dry skin:** The presence of flaky, scaly, or dry patches on the skin may indicate a problem that needs attention.
5. **Presence of external parasites:** Lice, mites, or other external parasites can cause feather loss and skin irritation. Look for tiny insects or their eggs on the feathers or skin.

Soothing skin problems:

Addressing skin problems and feather loss requires a comprehensive approach. Here are some strategies to help alleviate these issues:

1. **Regular health checks:** Conduct regular health checks on your chickens to identify problems early. Inspect their feathers, skin, and overall appearance, keeping an eye out for any abnormalities.
2. **Clean living environment**: Ensure that your chicken coop is clean, dry, and well-ventilated. Regularly remove waste and provide fresh bedding to prevent the buildup of bacteria or parasites that could contribute to skin issues.
3. **Nutritious diet:** Proper nutrition is crucial for maintaining healthy skin and feathers. Ensure your chickens have a balanced diet with adequate protein, vitamins, and minerals. Incorporate high-quality commercial feed and offer fresh fruits, vegetables, and supplements recommended for poultry.
4. **Parasite prevention and treatment:** Implement a regular parasite prevention program, including the use of appropriate treatments to control external parasites such as lice and mites. Consult with a veterinarian to determine the best products and methods for your chickens.
5. **Stress reduction:** Minimize stressors in your chickens' environment, as stress can contribute to skin problems. Provide ample space, comfortable roosting areas, and opportunities for exercise. Avoid overcrowding and sudden changes in their surroundings.
6. **Bathing and grooming:** Some chickens benefit from gentle bathing to clean their feathers and soothe their skin. Use lukewarm water and mild, poultry-safe shampoo or herbal rinses specifically designed for chickens. Gently dry them afterward to prevent chilling.
7. **Herbal remedies and supplements:** Certain herbs and supplements, such as calendula, chamomile, or essential oils, may have soothing effects on chicken skin. Consult with a veterinarian or poultry specialist to determine safe and effective options.
8. **Veterinary assistance:** If the skin problems persist or worsen despite your efforts, seek veterinary assistance. A professional can help diagnose and treat underlying conditions that

may be causing the issues.

Maintaining healthy skin and feathers is crucial for the overall well-being of your chickens. By observing any changes, implementing preventive measures, ensuring proper nutrition, and providing suitable treatments, you can address skin problems and feather loss in your flock effectively. Remember, the Chicken Health Bible is an ongoing learning process, so stay attentive to your chickens' needs and consult with professionals to ensure their optimal health and happiness.

Dizzy Chicken and Other Alarming Signs

The nervous system plays a vital role in the overall health and well-being of chickens. As poultry owners, it is crucial to be aware of the signs and symptoms of nervous system problems in our feathered friends. From dizziness to abnormal behaviors, understanding these alarming signs can help us react promptly and provide appropriate care. In this chapter of the Chicken Health Bible, we delve into the intricate world of the chicken's nervous system and explore how to respond to potential issues.

Chickens, like any living creatures, are susceptible to various nervous system disorders. While some conditions may arise due to genetic factors or pre-existing health conditions, others may be triggered by infections, injuries, or environmental factors. One of the most common indicators of a nervous system problem in chickens is dizziness. If you notice your chicken stumbling, falling, or experiencing difficulties maintaining balance, it could be a sign of an underlying issue.

Besides dizziness, there are several other alarming signs that may point towards nervous system problems in chickens. These signs include tremors or shaking, seizures, muscle weakness or paralysis, loss of coordination, abnormal behaviors such as aggression or fearfulness, and changes in vision or eye movements. It's important to note that these symptoms may vary depending on the specific disorder or condition affecting the nervous system.

When faced with a chicken displaying these alarming signs, it's essential to react promptly and provide appropriate care. The first step is to isolate the affected chicken from the rest of the flock to prevent the potential spread of infectious diseases or injuries. Next, consult a veterinarian who specializes in avian health to obtain an accurate diagnosis and develop a treatment plan.

To aid in diagnosing the issue, your veterinarian may conduct a thorough physical examination, review the chicken's medical history, and possibly recommend additional tests such as blood work, X-rays, or neurological evaluations. These diagnostic tools help map out the extent of the nervous system problem and provide valuable insights into the underlying cause.

The treatment approach for nervous system disorders in chickens varies depending on the specific condition and its severity. In some cases, medication may be prescribed to alleviate symptoms or manage underlying infections. Physical therapy or rehabilitation exercises may also be recommended to help chickens regain coordination and muscle strength. Additionally, ensuring a comfortable and stress-free environment for the affected chicken can contribute to their overall recovery.

Prevention is always better than cure when it comes to nervous system problems in chickens.

Maintaining good flock management practices, such as providing a clean and safe living environment, a balanced diet, and regular veterinary check-ups, can help minimize the risk of these issues. Additionally, keeping an eye on any changes in your chicken's behavior or physical appearance and addressing them promptly can prevent potential complications.

Being aware of the signs and symptoms of nervous system problems in chickens is essential for every poultry owner. Dizziness, tremors, abnormal behaviors, and other alarming signs can indicate underlying issues with the chicken's nervous system. Reacting promptly by isolating the affected chicken, consulting a veterinarian, and following their guidance is crucial for successful treatment and recovery. By mapping out these issues and taking appropriate action, we can ensure the well-being and health of our feathered companions.

Leg and Foot Issues

Keeping backyard chickens is a rewarding and enjoyable experience, but it also comes with the responsibility of ensuring their health and well-being. Chickens, like any living creatures, can experience leg and foot issues that may cause pain and discomfort. Understanding and addressing these problems promptly is crucial to maintain the overall health of your feathered friends. In this article, we'll zoom in on common leg and foot issues in chickens and discuss treatment options to help your chickens get back on their feet.

Bumblefoot:

Bumblefoot is a common condition in chickens characterized by a bacterial infection that affects the footpad. It often starts with a small cut or injury on the foot, which allows bacteria to enter and cause inflammation. The affected area becomes swollen, red, and may develop a black, scabby scab. To treat bumblefoot, you'll need to soak the foot in warm, Epsom salt water to help draw out infection. Then, carefully remove the scab, clean the wound, and apply an antibiotic ointment. In severe cases, your vet may need to perform surgery to remove the infected tissue.

Leg Mites:

Leg mites are tiny parasites that infest the legs of chickens, causing irritation, itching, and scaling of the skin. Infected birds may scratch excessively and develop scabs or crusty patches on their legs. To treat leg mites, you'll need to isolate the affected chicken, thoroughly clean the coop, and apply an appropriate mite treatment to the legs. It's important to follow the instructions carefully and repeat the treatment as necessary to eliminate the mites completely.

Leg Injuries:

Chickens can sustain leg injuries due to falls, predator attacks, or even getting their legs caught in wire fencing. Fractured or dislocated legs can be extremely painful and require immediate attention. If you suspect a leg injury, it's essential to separate the injured bird from the rest of the flock, provide a comfortable and quiet space, and consult a veterinarian. The vet will assess the injury and may recommend splinting, bandaging, or even surgery, depending on the severity of the condition.

Vitamin and Mineral Deficiencies:

Nutritional imbalances can contribute to leg and foot issues in chickens. Deficiencies in essential vitamins and minerals like calcium, vitamin D, and manganese can lead to weak bones, leg deformities, and conditions like rickets. To prevent such problems, ensure your chickens have access to a balanced diet that includes commercial poultry feed, fresh greens, and oyster shells for calcium supplementation. A poultry-specific vitamin and mineral supplement may also be recommended.

Gout:

Gout is a metabolic disorder that can affect chickens, causing swollen joints and discomfort. It is often caused by a diet high in purines, which are found in certain foods like meat scraps, organ meats, and some legumes. To manage gout, it's essential to provide a low-purine diet, consisting primarily of a balanced poultry feed and limited treats. Your vet may also prescribe medications to alleviate pain and reduce inflammation.

Remember, early detection and prompt treatment are essential when it comes to leg and foot issues in chickens. Regularly inspect your birds' legs and feet for any signs of redness, swelling, scabs, or limping. Maintaining a clean and well-maintained coop, offering a balanced diet, and providing ample space for exercise can significantly reduce the risk of leg and foot problems in your flock.

If you're uncertain about any leg or foot issue, it's always best to consult a poultry veterinarian for a proper diagnosis and guidance on treatment options. By being proactive in caring for your chickens' leg and foot health, you'll ensure they live a comfortable and active life as happy members of your backyard flock.

Chapter 9

Sick Chicks

Keeping your chicks healthy is crucial for their overall well-being and growth. In this chapter, we will discuss various aspects of chick health and provide guidance on how to address common issues that may arise. From spotting problems in newly hatched chicks to dealing with malformations and other concerns, this chapter aims to equip you with the knowledge to ensure the health of your flock.

Spotting Problems of the Newly Hatched:

When chicks first hatch, it's essential to closely observe them for any signs of problems. Here are some common issues to watch out for:

1. **Weakness or lethargy**: If a chick appears weak or unable to stand or move properly, it may indicate a problem. This could be due to an illness, nutritional deficiency, or physical injury during the hatching process.
2. **Abnormal feather development:** Chicks with abnormal feather growth or missing feathers may have underlying health issues. This could be a result of genetic factors, nutritional deficiencies, or external parasites.
3. **Difficulty breathing:** Chicks struggling to breathe or exhibiting rapid, labored breathing may be suffering from respiratory problems. Respiratory infections can spread quickly among a flock, so it's crucial to isolate affected birds and seek veterinary advice.

Finding Reasons for Chick Malformations:

Sometimes, newly hatched chicks may have malformations, which can vary in severity. Identifying the causes of these malformations is important for addressing the issue and preventing similar problems in the future. Here are a few common malformations and their potential causes:

1. **Curled toes:** Curled or crooked toes may result from genetic factors, nutritional

imbalances, or incubation issues such as improper humidity levels or excessive temperature fluctuations.
2. **Splayed legs:** Spraddled legs occur when a chick's legs splay out to the sides instead of standing straight. This condition can be caused by poor traction on slippery surfaces, vitamin deficiencies, or improper incubation conditions.

Straightening Spraddle Legs:

If you notice a chick with spraddle legs, it's essential to address the issue promptly to prevent long-term problems. Here's a simple method to straighten spraddle legs:

1. **Create a supportive brace:** Cut a small piece of adhesive medical tape or use a band-aid and place the chick's legs in a natural standing position, ensuring they are aligned correctly.
2. **Secure the brace:** Gently wrap the tape around the legs, creating a figure-eight shape that holds the legs in the correct position. Be careful not to wrap it too tightly, as this can restrict blood circulation.
3. **Monitor the chick:** Keep a close eye on the chick to ensure it can eat, drink, and move comfortably. Adjust the brace as necessary to accommodate the chick's growth.

Singing the Belly-Button Blues:

After hatching, some chicks may have an umbilical hernia, also known as a "belly-button" or "navel" hernia. This occurs when the chick's abdominal organs protrude through the weakened umbilical opening. If left untreated, the hernia can become a serious health issue. In such cases, it's best to consult a veterinarian for proper evaluation and treatment options.

Unpasting a Pasty Vent:

A pasty vent is a common condition in chicks, where droppings accumulate around the vent area, forming a blockage. This can prevent the chick from defecating properly, leading to discomfort and potential health problems. To resolve this issue:

1. **Prepare warm water:** Gently soak the chick's vent area in warm water for a few minutes. Ensure the water is not too hot to avoid scalding the chick.
2. **Gently clean the vent:** Using a soft cloth or cotton swab, gently remove the dried droppings from the vent area. Take care not to tug or injure the chick's delicate skin.
3. **Dry the chick:** After cleaning, pat the chick's vent area gently with a soft towel to remove excess moisture. Ensure the chick is warm and dry before returning it to its brooder.

By staying vigilant and addressing health concerns promptly, you can help ensure the well-being and vitality of your chicks. Remember, when in doubt or if issues persist, always seek professional advice from a veterinarian or experienced poultry expert. With proper care and attention, you can raise a healthy and thriving flock.

Problems of Growing Chickens

Raising chickens can be a rewarding experience, whether for meat or egg production. However, just like any living creatures, chickens are susceptible to various health issues. In this article, we will discuss three common problems that can affect growing chickens: respiratory problems, diarrhea in young chickens, and nervous system illnesses. Understanding these issues and their potential causes is essential for maintaining a healthy flock and ensuring their well-being.

Respiratory Problems:

Respiratory problems are a frequent concern among chicken farmers. These issues can manifest as coughing, sneezing, nasal discharge, or difficulty breathing. Respiratory infections can be caused by bacteria, viruses, fungi, or environmental factors such as poor ventilation or dust.

To prevent respiratory problems, it is crucial to maintain proper ventilation in chicken coops and ensure a clean and dry environment. Avoid overcrowding, as it can lead to increased stress and the spread of diseases. Vaccinations against common respiratory pathogens are available and can provide protection to the flock. If respiratory problems arise, consulting a veterinarian for diagnosis and appropriate treatment is recommended.

Diarrhea in Young Chickens:

Diarrhea is a common problem observed in young chickens, especially those raised for meat production. It can occur due to various reasons, such as bacterial or viral infections, dietary imbalances, stress, or parasitic infestations. Diarrhea can lead to dehydration and nutrient loss, negatively impacting the growth and development of chicks.

To manage diarrhea, it is essential to provide clean and uncontaminated water, as well as balanced and nutritious feed. Adequate hygiene practices, including regular cleaning of waterers and feeders, are crucial in preventing the spread of pathogens. In severe cases, isolating affected chicks and seeking veterinary advice may be necessary to identify the underlying cause and provide appropriate treatment.

Nervous System Illnesses in Young Chickens:

Nervous system illnesses can affect young chickens, leading to symptoms such as unsteady gait, tremors, paralysis, or abnormal behavior. These conditions can be caused by viral, bacterial, or parasitic infections, nutrient deficiencies, toxins, or genetic factors.

Prevention of nervous system illnesses involves proper biosecurity measures to limit exposure to infectious agents. A well-balanced diet, including essential vitamins and minerals, helps strengthen the immune system and reduce the risk of deficiencies. Vaccinations against common viral infections, such as Marek's disease, can provide protection against nervous system disorders. If any symptoms arise, consulting a veterinarian is crucial for proper diagnosis and appropriate treatment.

Maintaining the health of growing chickens is vital for their overall well-being and productivity.

Respiratory problems, diarrhea in young chickens, and nervous system illnesses are common challenges that chicken farmers may encounter. By implementing good husbandry practices, such as proper ventilation, hygiene, balanced nutrition, and preventive measures like vaccinations, many of these problems can be minimized or avoided altogether. Regular monitoring of the flock's health, prompt identification of any issues, and seeking professional advice when needed will contribute to the success of your chicken-raising endeavors. Remember, a healthy flock leads to happier and more productive chickens.

Chapter 10

Chicken Parasites

Welcome to Chapter 10 of the Chicken Health Bible! In this chapter, we will explore the fascinating and important topic of chicken parasites. As poultry owners, it is crucial to understand the various parasites that can affect our feathered friends and the potential risks they pose to their health.

Parasites are organisms that live on or inside another organism, known as the host, and depend on the host for survival. Unfortunately, chickens are susceptible to a range of parasites that can cause a variety of health issues if left untreated. These parasites can include mites, lice, fleas, ticks, worms, and more.

Throughout this chapter, we will delve into the characteristics, life cycles, and impact of these parasites on chickens. We will discuss the signs and symptoms of infestation, the potential consequences for your flock, and the necessary preventive measures and treatment options available.

Understanding the different types of chicken parasites is essential for maintaining a healthy and productive flock. Parasitic infestations can lead to decreased egg production, weight loss, anemia, skin irritation, feather damage, and even death in severe cases. By identifying and addressing parasitic issues promptly, we can prevent these negative outcomes and ensure the well-being of our chickens.

We will explore effective strategies for parasite prevention, including regular health checks, maintaining clean coops and surroundings, implementing biosecurity measures, and practicing good hygiene. Additionally, we will delve into treatment options such as topical treatments, dusting powders, oral medications, and natural remedies.

Remember, knowledge is the key to safeguarding your chickens' health. By familiarizing yourself with the signs, risks, and prevention methods related to chicken parasites, you will be well-equipped to provide the necessary care and protection for your flock.

So, let's dive into Chapter 10: Chicken Parasites and empower ourselves with the knowledge needed to ensure the health and happiness of our feathered companions!

Internal Parasites

Maintaining the health of chickens is essential for successful poultry farming. Unfortunately, internal parasites pose a significant threat to the well-being and productivity of chickens. In this comprehensive guide, we will explore three common types of internal parasites that affect chickens: coccidiosis, parasitic worms, and other less common infestations. By understanding the signs, prevention measures, and treatment options for these parasites, you can ensure the health and vitality of your chicken flock.

Coccidiosis:

Coccidiosis is a highly prevalent and economically significant parasitic disease caused by protozoa of the genus Eimeria. It affects the intestinal tract of chickens and can result in severe damage to the gut lining, leading to decreased nutrient absorption, poor growth, and increased susceptibility to other diseases.

Symptoms:

1. Diarrhea, sometimes with blood.
2. Decreased appetite and weight loss.
3. Dehydration and weakness.
4. Reduced egg production.
5. Increased mortality, especially in young birds.

Prevention and Control:

1. Maintain a clean and dry environment for chickens, regularly removing feces.
2. Provide good ventilation and reduce overcrowding.
3. Use anticoccidial medications or vaccines as preventive measures.
4. Avoid introducing infected birds or contaminated equipment to your flock.
5. Implement proper biosecurity protocols.

Treatment:

1. Consult a veterinarian for diagnosis and treatment options.
2. Administer anticoccidial drugs as prescribed.
3. Isolate and treat affected birds to prevent further spread.
4. Follow withdrawal periods for medication to avoid residues in poultry products.

Parasitic Worms:

Parasitic worms, such as roundworms (nematodes) and tapeworms (cestodes), are common internal parasites that affect chickens worldwide. These worms can infect various organs, including the intestines, crop, esophagus, and trachea, causing various health issues.

Symptoms:

1. Poor growth and reduced feed efficiency.
2. Pale comb and wattles due to anemia.
3. Increased appetite combined with weight loss.
4. Diarrhea or abnormal feces.
5. Dull feathers and reduced egg production.
6. Lethargy and weakness.

Prevention and Control:

1. Practice regular deworming using appropriate anthelmintic drugs.
2. Maintain good hygiene and sanitation in the coop and surroundings.
3. Avoid free-ranging chickens in areas prone to contamination.
4. Rotate pasture areas regularly to reduce parasite burden.
5. Quarantine new birds before introducing them to the flock.

Treatment:

1. Consult a veterinarian for accurate diagnosis and appropriate deworming drugs.
2. Administer dewormers according to the manufacturer's instructions.
3. Follow withdrawal periods before consuming eggs or meat from treated chickens.
4. Regularly monitor and retest the flock to evaluate the effectiveness of treatment.

Other Internal Parasites:

Besides coccidiosis and parasitic worms, chickens can be affected by other internal parasites, although they are less common. These include:

1. **Gapeworms (Syngamus trachea):** These worms reside in the trachea and can cause respiratory distress, including gasping, coughing, and choking.
2. **Hairworms (Capillaria spp.):** These thin, thread-like worms infest the digestive tract, leading to weight loss, anemia, and diarrhea.
3. **Heterakis worms (Heterakis gallinarum):** These worms are commonly found in the cecum and can transmit the parasite Histomonas meleagridis, causing blackhead disease in turkeys and chickens.

Prevention, Control, and Treatment:

1. Similar preventive measures and treatment strategies as for coccidiosis and parasitic worms apply.
2. Accurate diagnosis through fecal examinations is crucial to identify the specific parasites and determine appropriate treatment options.
3. Consult a veterinarian for guidance on preventive measures, diagnosis, and treatment.

Internal parasites, including coccidiosis, parasitic worms, and other less common infestations, can significantly impact the health and productivity of chickens. By implementing effective preventive measures, maintaining good hygiene, and consulting with a veterinarian, when necessary, you can minimize the risk and ensure the well-being of your chicken flock. Regular monitoring, proper diagnosis, and prompt treatment are key to keeping your chickens healthy and maintaining optimal production in your poultry operation. Remember, a proactive approach to internal parasite control is essential for maintaining a thriving chicken flock.

External Parasites

In the world of chicken health and care, external parasites pose a significant threat to the well-being and productivity of poultry. These tiny creatures, such as poultry lice, mites, chiggers, fleas, and bedbugs, can wreak havoc on a chicken's health and lead to various issues. Therefore, it is essential for chicken owners and farmers to be aware of these external parasites, understand their impact, and learn effective prevention and treatment strategies. In this comprehensive guide, we will delve into the world of external parasites, focusing on poultry lice, mites, and other common pests.

Poultry Lice:

1. **Description and Life Cycle:** Poultry lice are wingless insects that infest chickens, causing severe discomfort and health problems. They are typically divided into two types: biting lice and sucking lice. Biting lice feed on feathers and skin debris, while sucking lice consume blood. Understanding their life cycle and habits is crucial for effective management.
2. **Symptoms and Impact on Chickens:** Lice infestation can lead to a range of symptoms, including feather loss, irritation, itching, decreased egg production, anemia, and stunted growth. These parasites can quickly multiply and spread to other birds in the flock, exacerbating the problems.
3. **Prevention and Treatment:** Preventing lice infestation involves maintaining proper coop hygiene, regularly inspecting birds for signs of lice, and implementing effective biosecurity measures. Treatment options include dusting birds with poultry-friendly insecticides, applying natural remedies, and ensuring the coop is thoroughly cleaned and treated.

Mites:

1. **Common Types of Mites:** Mites are another type of external parasites that commonly affect poultry. Common types include the Northern fowl mite, red mite, scaly leg mite, and the depluming mite. Each mite species presents unique challenges and requires specific management techniques.
2. **Symptoms and Impact on Chickens:** Mite infestation can cause severe skin irritation, feather loss, anemia, decreased egg production, and compromised immune function. It is crucial to identify the symptoms early to prevent the mites from spreading and causing further damage.
3. **Prevention and Treatment:** Preventing mite infestations involves maintaining a clean and

dry environment, regularly inspecting birds for signs of mites, and using appropriate dust baths or diatomaceous earth. Treatment options include topical insecticides, natural remedies, and regular coop cleaning and disinfection.

Chiggers, Fleas, and Bedbugs:

1. **Chiggers:** Chiggers are tiny mites that can cause intense itching and irritation in chickens. They usually infest the legs, vent area, and underbelly of birds.
2. **Fleas:** Fleas are small, wingless insects that can transmit diseases to chickens. They cause itching, discomfort, and can impact a chicken's overall health.
3. **Bedbugs:** Bed Bugs are nocturnal insects that primarily infect chicken coops. While they don't directly harm chickens, their presence can lead to stress, discomfort, and sleep disturbances.

Prevention and treatment strategies for chiggers, fleas, and bedbugs often overlap with those for lice and mites. Maintaining good coop hygiene, practicing regular inspections, and using appropriate insecticides or natural remedies can help control these pests.

External parasites pose a significant threat to the health and productivity of poultry. Understanding the characteristics, symptoms, and management strategies for poultry lice, mites, chiggers, fleas, and bedbugs is essential for every chicken owner and farmer. By implementing preventative measures, regularly monitoring the flock, and employing effective treatment methods, chicken enthusiasts can ensure the well-being and vitality of their feathered friends. Remember, a proactive approach to managing external parasites will help maintain a healthy and thriving chicken flock.

Chapter 11

Diseases Caused By Protozoa

In the Chicken Health Bible, it is crucial to understand and address the various diseases that can affect chickens. Protozoa are microscopic single-celled organisms that can cause several diseases in poultry, including chickens. These diseases can significantly impact the health, welfare, and productivity of chicken flocks. This chapter focuses on the diseases caused by protozoa in chickens, providing an overview of the most common protozoal infections, their symptoms, prevention, and treatment strategies.

Coccidiosis:

Coccidiosis is one of the most prevalent protozoan diseases in chickens. It is caused by several species of the protozoan parasite Eimeria. The parasites primarily affect the intestinal tract of chickens, leading to severe damage to the gut lining and subsequent health issues. Common symptoms of coccidiosis include diarrhea, decreased appetite, weight loss, dehydration, and poor growth. Proper sanitation, biosecurity measures, and strategic use of anticoccidial drugs can help prevent and control coccidiosis.

Histomoniasis (Blackhead Disease):

Histomoniasis, commonly known as Blackhead disease, is caused by the protozoan parasite Histomonas meleagridis. This disease affects not only chickens but also turkeys and other game birds. The parasites are transmitted by a common poultry nematode, Heterakis gallinarum, which acts as a carrier. Infected birds may show symptoms such as depression, reduced appetite, weight loss, diarrhea, and a characteristic black discoloration of the head region. Strict biosecurity, proper management practices, and deworming programs can help prevent Histomoniasis.

Trichomoniasis:

Trichomoniasis, caused by the protozoan parasite Trichomonas gallinae, primarily affects the upper digestive tract of chickens. This disease is often characterized by the presence of yellowish or greenish frothy droppings and the formation of cheesy masses in the mouth, throat, and esophagus. Infected birds may also exhibit difficulty in swallowing, reduced appetite, weight loss, and lethargy. Good hygiene, strict biosecurity, and regular monitoring are essential for preventing and controlling Trichomoniasis.

Toxoplasmosis:

Toxoplasmosis is caused by the protozoan parasite Toxoplasma gondii, which can infect various warm-blooded animals, including chickens. Chickens become infected through ingestion of oocysts shed by infected cats or consumption of contaminated feed or water. While chickens typically show no clinical signs of infection, the parasite can be transmitted to humans through the consumption of undercooked or raw chicken meat and pose a health risk, especially to pregnant women. Proper hygiene, preventing access to cats, and thorough cooking of poultry products can reduce the risk of Toxoplasma infection.

Giardiasis:

Giardiasis is caused by the protozoan parasite Giardia spp. It primarily affects the small intestine of chickens. Infected birds may display symptoms such as diarrhea, weight loss, decreased appetite, and poor feather quality. Giardia infections can occur in crowded or unsanitary conditions, making good management practices, clean drinking water, and regular sanitation crucial for prevention and control.

Protozoal diseases can have a significant impact on the health and productivity of chicken flocks. Understanding the diseases caused by protozoa, their symptoms, prevention, and treatment is essential for poultry farmers and caretakers. By implementing good management practices, practicing strict biosecurity measures, and utilizing appropriate preventive and therapeutic measures, the risks associated with protozoal infections can be minimized. Regular monitoring and veterinary consultation are recommended to ensure the health and well-being of chickens and to maintain a successful poultry operation.

Chapter 12

Diseases Caused By Bacteria And Viruses

Diseases Caused By Bacteria

Welcome to Chapter 12 of the Chicken Health Bible! In this chapter, we will explore a crucial aspect of chicken health—diseases caused by bacteria. Bacteria are microscopic organisms that can pose significant threats to the well-being of your flock. Understanding these diseases and their prevention is essential for maintaining a healthy and thriving chicken population.

Bacterial infections can affect chickens of all ages and breeds, and their consequences can range from mild discomfort to severe illness and even death. The immune system of chickens is well-equipped to combat many bacterial invaders, but certain factors, such as stress, overcrowding, poor nutrition, or unsanitary conditions, can weaken their defenses, making them more susceptible to infections.

In this chapter, we will delve into the most common bacterial diseases that afflict chickens, including symptoms, transmission methods, and effective prevention strategies. We will discuss diseases like Avian Cholera, Infectious Coryza, Fowl Typhoid, and many more. Each disease will be examined in detail, providing you with a comprehensive understanding of the pathogens responsible, their impact on chicken health, and the appropriate treatment options.

Furthermore, we will explore the importance of maintaining good biosecurity practices to prevent the introduction and spread of bacterial diseases. You will learn about proper sanitation measures, effective vaccination protocols, and ways to minimize stress in your flock—all of which play a vital role in safeguarding your chickens from harmful bacteria.

By the end of this chapter, you will have a thorough understanding of the diseases caused by bacteria in chickens and the proactive measures you can take to keep your flock healthy and thriving. Armed with this knowledge, you will be better equipped to recognize the signs of bacterial infections, implement appropriate prevention strategies, and ensure the overall well-being of your chickens.

So, let's dive into Chapter 12 and unlock the secrets to effectively managing and preventing diseases caused by bacteria in your flock. Your commitment to chicken health and welfare will undoubtedly lead to happier, healthier, and more productive chickens.

Diseases caused by bacteria:

Avian Intestinal Spirochetosis:

Avian intestinal spirochetosis is a bacterial disease that affects the intestinal tract of chickens. It is caused by certain species of spirochetes, spiral-shaped bacteria. The disease can lead to reduced feed efficiency, diarrhea, weight loss, and sometimes death.

Avian Tuberculosis:

Avian tuberculosis, also known as avian mycobacteriosis, is a chronic bacterial infection caused by Mycobacterium avium. This disease can affect various organs in the chicken's body, including the liver, spleen, and intestines. It can result in poor growth, reduced egg production, and increased mortality.

Colibacillosis (E. coli Infections):

Colibacillosis is a bacterial infection caused by Escherichia coli (E. coli) bacteria. Chickens can become infected through contaminated water, feed, or environments. The disease manifests in different forms, including respiratory, enteric, and septicemic forms. Colibacillosis can lead to diarrhea, respiratory distress, swollen joints, and high mortality rates.

Fowl Cholera:

Fowl cholera is a highly contagious bacterial disease caused by Pasteurella multocida. It affects various species of birds, including chickens. The disease can manifest as acute or chronic forms and commonly affects the respiratory system. Symptoms include swollen wattles, difficulty breathing, fever, and sudden death.

Infectious Coryza:

Infectious coryza is a bacterial respiratory disease caused by Avibacterium paragallinarum. It primarily affects chickens but can also infect other poultry species. The disease spreads through direct contact or respiratory secretions. Common symptoms include facial swelling, nasal discharge, sneezing, and reduced egg production.

Mycoplasmosis:

Mycoplasmosis is a bacterial disease caused by Mycoplasma gallisepticum and Mycoplasma synoviae. It affects multiple systems in chickens, including the respiratory, reproductive, and musculoskeletal systems. The disease can cause respiratory distress, coughing, swollen joints, reduced egg production, and increased susceptibility to secondary infections.

Necrotic Enteritis:

Necrotic enteritis is a bacterial disease caused by Clostridium perfringens, specifically certain strains that produce toxins. It affects the intestinal tract of chickens, leading to necrosis and inflammation of the gut lining. Symptoms include diarrhea, reduced growth rate, and increased mortality, particularly in birds with compromised gut health.

Pullorum Disease and Fowl Typhoid:

Pullorum disease and fowl typhoid are bacterial infections caused by Salmonella bacteria. Pullorum disease primarily affects young chicks, while fowl typhoid affects older birds. These diseases are characterized by general systemic infection, including high mortality rates, reduced growth, and reproductive problems.

Chapter 12 of the "Chicken Health Bible" explores diseases caused by bacteria and viruses, shedding light on their symptoms, causes, and management strategies. By equipping chicken owners with knowledge and resources, the aim is to promote the overall health and well-being of chickens, leading to sustainable and successful poultry farming practices.

Diseases Caused by Viruses

Keeping chickens healthy is crucial for successful poultry farming and backyard chicken enthusiasts. One of the most significant threats to chicken health is viral diseases. Viruses are microscopic infectious agents that can cause a range of illnesses in chickens, affecting their overall well-being and productivity. In this comprehensive guide, we will discuss some common viral diseases that can afflict chickens, their symptoms, prevention, and potential treatments.

Avian Encephalomyelitis:

Avian encephalomyelitis is a viral disease that affects the central nervous system of chickens. It can cause various symptoms, including tremors, paralysis, and a decrease in egg production. The virus is typically transmitted through contaminated feed or water. Vaccination is an effective preventive measure against avian encephalomyelitis.

Avian Influenza:

Avian influenza, also known as bird flu, is a highly contagious viral disease that affects birds, including chickens. It can cause severe respiratory distress, decreased egg production, and high mortality rates. Some strains of avian influenza viruses can also infect humans, posing a potential public health risk. Preventive measures include strict biosecurity practices and vaccination in certain regions.

Chicken Infectious Anemia:

Chicken infectious anemia is caused by a small DNA virus and primarily affects young chickens. It leads to anemia, immunosuppression, and poor growth. The virus is mainly transmitted vertically from infected hens to their offspring. Strict biosecurity measures and maintaining a clean environment can help prevent the disease.

Fowl Pox:

Fowl pox is a viral disease characterized by the formation of wart-like lesions on the unfeathered parts of a chicken's body, such as the comb, wattles, and legs. It can cause reduced appetite, weight loss, and decreased egg production. The virus is transmitted through direct contact with infected birds or contaminated surfaces. Vaccination is an effective preventive measure against fowl pox.

Infectious Bronchitis:

Infectious bronchitis is a highly contagious respiratory disease caused by the infectious bronchitis virus (IBV). It can lead to respiratory distress, coughing, sneezing, nasal discharge, and decreased egg production. The virus spreads through respiratory secretions and can survive in the environment for several weeks. Vaccination and strict biosecurity practices are crucial in preventing infectious bronchitis.

Infectious Bursal Disease:

Infectious bursal disease (IBD), also known as Gumboro disease, primarily affects young chickens and targets the immune system. It can cause immunosuppression, leading to increased susceptibility to other infections. The virus is transmitted through contaminated feces, water, and equipment. Vaccination is essential to prevent IBD.

Infectious Laryngotracheitis:

Infectious laryngotracheitis (ILT) is a respiratory disease characterized by severe inflammation of the larynx and trachea. It can cause respiratory distress, coughing, sneezing, and bloody mucus discharge. The virus spreads through respiratory secretions and can persist in the environment. Vaccination and strict biosecurity measures are important for preventing ILT.

Lymphoid Leukosis:

Lymphoid leukosis is a viral disease that affects chickens, causing cancerous tumors in various organs, including the liver, spleen, and kidneys. The virus is transmitted through contaminated eggs or direct contact with infected birds. Strict biosecurity practices, culling infected birds, and testing breeding flocks can help control lymphoid leukosis.

Marek's Disease:

Marek's disease is a highly contagious viral disease that affects chickens, primarily between the ages of 3 and 25 weeks. It can cause paralysis, tumors in various organs, and immunosuppression. The virus spreads through dander, feather follicles, and contaminated environments. Vaccination is the most effective preventive measure against Marek's disease.

Newcastle Disease:

Newcastle disease, also known as avian paramyxovirus, is a highly contagious viral disease that affects various bird species, including chickens. It can cause respiratory distress, nervous system disorders, and high mortality rates. The virus spreads through respiratory secretions and feces. Vaccination and strict biosecurity practices are crucial in preventing Newcastle disease.

Understanding the viral diseases that can affect chickens is essential for maintaining their health and productivity. Implementing strict biosecurity measures, practicing proper sanitation, and following vaccination protocols are key preventive strategies. Regular monitoring and consultation with a veterinarian can help identify and manage viral diseases effectively, ensuring the overall well-being of your chickens and the success of your poultry farming endeavors.

Chapter 13

Fungus And Mystery Diseases Fungal Infections

Welcome to Chapter 13 of the Chicken Health Bible, where we delve into the intriguing world of fungal infections and their impact on chicken health. Fungi are microorganisms that can cause a wide range of diseases in chickens, often leading to significant challenges for poultry farmers and backyard chicken enthusiasts alike. These mysterious diseases can manifest in various ways, affecting the respiratory, digestive, or integumentary systems of our feathered friends.

In this chapter, we will explore the different types of fungal infections that can afflict chickens and examine their symptoms, causes, and potential treatments. We will shed light on the fascinating world of fungal pathogens and their life cycles, helping you understand how these organisms thrive and spread among your flock.

Understanding the signs and symptoms of fungal infections is crucial for early detection and effective management. We will discuss the common indicators of fungal diseases in chickens, including respiratory distress, skin lesions, abnormal feather growth, decreased egg production, and more. By recognizing these symptoms, you will be better equipped to take swift action and implement appropriate treatment measures.

Furthermore, we will explore the factors that contribute to the development and spread of fungal infections in chicken flocks. From environmental conditions to dietary imbalances and poor hygiene practices, we will uncover the risk factors that can increase the likelihood of fungal outbreaks. By addressing these underlying causes, you can minimize the chances of your chickens falling prey to these insidious infections.

Prevention is always better than cure, and we will provide you with practical strategies to safeguard your flock from fungal infections. From proper biosecurity measures to maintaining clean and dry living environments, we will equip you with the knowledge and tools needed to create a healthy and disease-resistant habitat for your chickens.

Lastly, we will explore the available treatment options for fungal infections in chickens, including antifungal medications, natural remedies, and supportive care. We will guide you through the process of diagnosing and treating these infections, highlighting the importance of veterinary advice and appropriate medication administration.

By the end of this chapter, you will have a comprehensive understanding of fungal infections in chickens, empowering you to protect your flock from these mysterious diseases. Whether you are a seasoned poultry farmer or a backyard chicken enthusiast, the knowledge gained from this chapter will be invaluable in maintaining the health and well-being of your feathered companions.

So let's embark on this fascinating journey into the realm of fungus and mystery diseases, as we uncover the secrets of fungal infections and their impact on chicken health in Chapter 13 of the Chicken Health Bible.

Molds and Yeasts

Maintaining the health of chickens is crucial for successful poultry farming. However, various factors, including environmental conditions, nutrition, and microbial infections, can impact their well-being. In this comprehensive guide, we will focus on three common fungal infections that affect chickens: Brooder pneumonia (Aspergillosis), Candidiasis (Thrush), and Ringworm (Favus). Understanding these conditions will help poultry farmers identify, prevent, and treat these ailments effectively.

Brooder Pneumonia (Aspergillosis):

Brooder pneumonia, also known as Aspergillosis, is a respiratory disease caused by the mold Aspergillus. It primarily affects young chicks and can be fatal if left untreated. The mold thrives in warm and damp environments, such as poorly ventilated brooder houses or contaminated bedding materials. Chickens may contract brooder pneumonia by inhaling spores or ingesting mold-contaminated feed.

- **Symptoms:** The symptoms of brooder pneumonia include labored breathing, coughing, nasal discharge, reduced appetite, weight loss, and lethargy. Affected chicks may exhibit gasping or open-mouthed breathing, indicating severe respiratory distress.
- **Prevention and Treatment:** To prevent brooder pneumonia, maintain proper ventilation and cleanliness in brooder houses. Avoid using damp bedding materials and regularly clean and disinfect feeders, waterers, and housing areas. Provide chicks with a clean and dry environment. Treatment typically involves antifungal medications prescribed by a veterinarian. Isolating infected birds is crucial to prevent the spread of the disease.

Candidiasis (Thrush):

Candidiasis, commonly known as Thrush, is a fungal infection caused by the yeast Candida albicans. It affects the digestive tract of chickens, particularly the crop and the gizzard. Candida yeast exists naturally in the digestive system, but certain conditions, such as stress, poor nutrition, or the prolonged use of antibiotics, can lead to an overgrowth, causing an infection.

- **Symptoms:** The symptoms of candidiasis include white or yellowish cheesy plaques in the mouth and throat, reduced appetite, weight loss, diarrhea, dehydration, and general weakness. In severe cases, the yeast infection can spread to other organs, leading to systemic candidiasis.
- **Prevention and Treatment:** Maintaining a balanced diet and avoiding prolonged antibiotic use can help prevent candidiasis. Regularly monitor and clean the chicken's drinking and feeding equipment to reduce the risk of contamination. Treatment involves administering antifungal medication as prescribed by a veterinarian. Good hygiene practices and proper nutrition are essential for successful recovery.

Ringworm (Favus):

Ringworm, scientifically known as Favus, is a highly contagious fungal infection caused by several species of fungi, including Trichophyton and Microsporum. It primarily affects the skin, feathers, and occasionally the beak of chickens. Ringworm can spread rapidly among birds in crowded and unsanitary conditions.

- **Symptoms:** Infected chickens develop circular or irregular lesions on the skin, particularly around the head, neck, and legs. These lesions appear crusty, scaly, and may lead to feather loss or beak deformities. Affected birds may exhibit itching, restlessness, and self-inflicted injuries from excessive scratching.
- **Prevention and Treatment:** Preventing ringworm involves maintaining a clean and dry environment, avoiding overcrowding, and providing adequate ventilation. Regularly inspect and quarantine new birds before introducing them to the flock. Treatment includes topical antifungal ointments or sprays, as well as systemic antifungal medications, depending on the severity of the infection. Prompt and appropriate treatment can prevent the spread of ringworm to other birds.

Understanding the common fungal infections that can affect chickens, such as brooder pneumonia, candidiasis, and ringworm, is crucial for poultry farmers. By implementing proper preventive measures, maintaining good hygiene practices, and promptly treating affected birds, farmers can protect the overall health and well-being of their flocks. Regular monitoring, seeking veterinary guidance when necessary, and providing optimal nutrition will help ensure the longevity and productivity of chickens in poultry farming operations.

Other Diseases with Mysterious Causes

The health and well-being of chickens are of paramount importance for poultry farmers. While many diseases affecting chickens have well-established causes, there are certain conditions that continue to baffle experts due to their mysterious origins. In this article, we delve into several enigmatic poultry diseases: broiler breakdowns, bumblefoot, crop problems (sour crop and impactions), gout, kidney stones, and misfires of the reproductive tract. Join us as we explore these perplexing conditions and discuss potential factors that may contribute to their development.

Broiler Breakdowns:

Broiler breakdowns refer to a phenomenon where broiler chickens, bred specifically for rapid growth and high meat production, suffer from musculoskeletal issues, leading to lameness and reduced mobility. While the precise cause of broiler breakdowns is not fully understood, genetic factors, nutrition, and management practices are thought to play a role. Breeding for rapid growth has resulted in chickens with disproportionately large body weight relative to their skeletal structure, potentially leading to stress on their legs and joints.

Bumblefoot (Pododermatitis):

Bumblefoot is a condition characterized by inflammation and infection of the footpad in chickens. It presents as a swollen, painful lesion that can progress to abscess formation. The exact cause of bumblefoot is often unknown, but it is believed to be associated with trauma to the footpad, poor litter quality, inappropriate flooring surfaces, and high body weight. Bacteria, such as Staphylococcus aureus, often contribute to the infection. Implementing proper flock management, maintaining clean housing conditions, and providing suitable flooring surfaces can help reduce the incidence of bumblefoot.

Crop Problems:

Sour Crop and Impactions: Crop problems, including sour crop and impactions, involve issues with the chicken's crop, which is the enlarged part of the esophagus responsible for temporary food storage. Sour crop occurs when the crop becomes distended and filled with a foul-smelling, fermenting mass of undigested food. Impactions, on the other hand, occur when the crop becomes impacted with material that cannot pass through the digestive system. The exact causes of these conditions are not always clear but may be associated with bacterial or fungal infections, nutritional imbalances, or obstructions. Proper diet, feed management, and ensuring access to clean water are crucial for preventing crop problems.

Gout and Kidney Stones:

Gout is a metabolic disorder characterized by the deposition of uric acid crystals in the joints of chickens, leading to painful inflammation and swelling. Kidney stones, or urate nephrolithiasis, occur when urate crystals accumulate in the kidneys. The precise causes of gout and kidney stones in chickens remain elusive, but genetic factors, imbalanced diets, dehydration, and impaired kidney function may contribute. Avoiding excessive dietary protein and ensuring adequate hydration are essential in managing and preventing these conditions.

Misfires of the Reproductive Tract:

Misfires of the reproductive tract encompass various disorders affecting the reproductive health of chickens. These disorders can lead to abnormalities in egg production, fertility, and hatchability. The causes of reproductive tract misfires can be multifactorial, including genetic factors, hormonal imbalances, infectious agents, nutritional deficiencies, and stress. Maintaining optimal environmental conditions, providing a balanced diet, and regular veterinary monitoring can aid in minimizing reproductive tract issues.

While many poultry diseases have identifiable causes, some conditions in chickens continue to perplex researchers and poultry farmers. Broiler breakdowns, bumblefoot, crop problems, gout, kidney stones, and reproductive tract misfires are among the enigmatic diseases that challenge our understanding. By further investigating the potential factors contributing to these conditions and implementing appropriate preventive measures, we can improve the overall health and well-being of chickens and ensure a more sustainable and successful poultry industry.

Chapter 14

Flock Management And Accidents

Welcome to Chapter 14 of the Chicken Health Bible, where we delve into the important topic of flock management and accidents. In order to maintain a healthy and thriving chicken flock, it is crucial to have a solid understanding of effective flock management techniques and to be prepared for potential accidents that can occur in your poultry operation.

This chapter aims to equip you with the knowledge and strategies necessary to manage your flock efficiently and minimize the risk of accidents. Whether you are a novice poultry keeper or an experienced farmer, the information provided here will help you ensure the well-being and productivity of your chickens.

Flock management involves various aspects, including housing, nutrition, disease prevention, and biosecurity. We will explore each of these areas in detail, offering practical tips and guidelines to help you create an optimal environment for your birds. From providing adequate housing and ventilation to implementing a balanced diet, you will learn how to promote the overall health and welfare of your flock.

Accidents can happen in any poultry operation, and being prepared for them is essential. We will discuss common accidents that can occur in a chicken flock, such as predator attacks, diseases outbreaks, and environmental hazards. Understanding the signs and symptoms of these incidents will enable you to take prompt action and minimize the impact on your flock.

Furthermore, we will provide guidance on emergency preparedness and first aid for chickens. Having a basic understanding of first aid techniques and knowing how to handle emergency situations can make a significant difference in saving the lives of your birds.

By the end of this chapter, you will have a comprehensive understanding of flock management practices and be better equipped to handle accidents that may arise. Remember, proactive and diligent management is the key to maintaining a healthy and thriving chicken flock.

So, let's delve into Chapter 14 and explore the world of flock management and accidents in the Chicken Health Bible. Get ready to enhance your knowledge and skills to create a safe and flourishing environment for your feathered friends!

Defending Against Predators

In the realm of chicken keeping, one of the primary concerns for poultry owners is the safety and well-being of their flock. Predators pose a significant threat to chickens, and effective defense strategies are crucial to ensure the health and security of these birds. When it comes to safeguarding your chickens against predators, a two-pronged approach involving the air attack and ground assault can be highly effective. This article will delve into both methods and provide insights into protecting your flock in the context of the Chicken Health Bible.

The Air Attack:

Predatory birds, such as hawks and eagles, are formidable adversaries that can swoop down on unsuspecting chickens. To defend against aerial predators, there are several measures you can take:

1. **Covered Runs and Enclosures:** Creating a covered run or enclosure for your chickens can be an excellent line of defense against airborne threats. These structures can be constructed using sturdy fencing and covered with netting or wire mesh to prevent predatory birds from reaching the chickens.
2. **Overhead Netting:** Installing overhead netting over the chicken yard can act as an additional barrier against aerial predators. Ensure that the netting is securely attached to prevent any gaps or openings that could allow access to the chickens.
3. **Roosting Covers:** Provide your chickens with covered roosting areas where they can seek shelter and protection from aerial attacks. Constructing covered roosting bars or installing enclosed roosting boxes can give chickens a safe haven during times of vulnerability, such as dusk and dawn when predatory birds are most active.
4. **Visual Deterrents:** Utilize visual deterrents like reflective surfaces, windsocks, or scarecrows near the chicken coop and run. These can startle predatory birds and deter them from approaching, reducing the likelihood of an attack.

The Ground Assault:

Predators that operate on the ground, such as foxes, raccoons, weasels, snakes, and even domestic pets like dogs, pose a significant threat to chickens. Employing effective strategies to defend against ground-based predators is essential for ensuring the safety of your flock:

1. **Secure Fencing:** Establishing a secure perimeter around the chicken coop and run is vital.

Use sturdy fencing materials that extend below ground level to prevent burrowing predators from gaining access. The fence should also be tall enough to deter predators from jumping over it.

2. **Electric Fencing:** Installing electric fencing can be an effective deterrent against predators. When properly installed, it delivers a harmless but startling shock to any creature that comes into contact with it, dissuading them from attempting to breach the enclosure.
3. **Predator-Proof Coop Design:** Constructing a predator-proof coop is of utmost importance. Ensure that all openings, including doors, windows, and vents, are securely covered with heavy-gauge wire mesh. Reinforce any weak points or gaps in the coop structure to prevent predators from gaining entry.
4. **Nighttime Security:** Many predators are nocturnal, making nighttime security measures crucial. Close the coop securely at night and ensure that all access points, such as windows and vents, are tightly shut. Consider using automatic coop doors that can be programmed to open and close at specific times, providing an added layer of protection.
5. **Guard Animals:** Employing guard animals, such as dogs or geese, can help deter predators. Trained livestock guardian dogs have a natural instinct to protect livestock, while geese are known for their loud honking and territorial nature, which can discourage intruders.

By combining these air attack and ground assault strategies, you can create a formidable defense system to protect your chickens against a wide range of predators. Remember, vigilance and proactive measures are key to ensuring the safety and well-being of your flock. Consult resources like the Chicken Health Bible for additional information on predator identification, prevention, and treatment to strengthen your defense strategies and maintain a healthy and thriving flock.

Flock-Mate Persecution or Cannibalism

Flock-mate persecution and cannibalism are distressing behaviors observed in chickens that can have significant consequences for flock health and productivity. These behaviors involve aggressive pecking, feather pecking, and even cannibalism among flock members. Understanding the causes behind these behaviors and implementing preventive measures are crucial for maintaining the well-being of chickens and ensuring a productive and harmonious flock. In this article, we will explore the causes of flock-mate persecution and cannibalism in chickens and discuss strategies to prevent and correct these behaviors.

Causes of Flock-Mate Persecution and Cannibalism:

Several factors contribute to the development of flock-mate persecution and cannibalism in chickens. It is important to identify and address these underlying causes to effectively prevent and correct these behaviors. Some common causes include:

1. **Overcrowding:** Insufficient space within the chicken coop or run can lead to stress, frustration, and heightened aggression among flock members.

2. **Boredom and Lack of Environmental Enrichment:** Chickens are naturally curious and social animals. Lack of stimulation, such as environmental enrichment, opportunities for foraging, or access to dust baths, can result in increased aggression.
3. **Nutritional Deficiencies:** Inadequate nutrition, particularly deficiencies in certain vitamins or minerals, can lead to abnormal behaviors in chickens. Imbalances in the diet can also contribute to feather pecking and cannibalism.
4. **Genetic Predisposition:** Some chicken breeds or strains may be more prone to aggressive behavior or have a higher likelihood of engaging in flock-mate persecution or cannibalism.

Prevention and Correction Strategies:

To prevent and correct flock-mate persecution and cannibalism behaviors, a multi-faceted approach should be employed. Here are some strategies to consider:

1. **Provide Sufficient Space:** Ensure that the chicken coop and run have ample space for the number of birds in the flock. Providing enough room allows chickens to establish a social hierarchy and reduces competition for resources.
2. **Environmental Enrichment:** Offer a variety of environmental enrichment options, such as perches, toys, and objects for pecking, to keep chickens mentally stimulated and engaged. This helps prevent boredom and aggressive behaviors.
3. **Balanced Nutrition:** Provide a well-balanced and nutritionally complete diet for chickens. Consult with a poultry nutritionist or veterinarian to ensure that the feed meets the specific nutritional requirements of the flock.
4. **Avoid Overcrowding:** Avoid overcrowding by maintaining appropriate stocking densities. Adequate space reduces stress and minimizes aggressive interactions between chickens.
5. **Beak Trimming:** In severe cases where cannibalism persists despite preventive measures, beak trimming may be necessary. This procedure, when performed by a professional, involves the removal of the sharp tip of the beak to minimize injuries from pecking.
6. **Behavioral Modification:** Observe the flock closely and identify aggressive individuals. Remove or isolate aggressive birds temporarily to prevent them from causing harm to others. Gradual reintroduction may be attempted once their behavior improves.
7. **Distractions and Diversion:** Offer distractions in the form of hanging treats, pecking blocks, or specially designed toys to redirect aggressive behavior and provide an outlet for pecking tendencies.
8. **Anti-Pecking Sprays or Lotions:** Certain sprays or lotions can be applied to the feathers of targeted birds to deter pecking and cannibalistic behaviors. These products usually have an unpleasant taste or odor that discourages further aggression.
9. **Monitor and Seek Veterinary Advice:** Regularly monitor the flock for signs of aggression, feather damage, or injuries. If the problem persists or worsens, consult a veterinarian experienced in poultry health for further guidance and potential medical interventions.

Flock-mate persecution and cannibalism are detrimental behaviors that can negatively impact chicken health and productivity. By understanding the underlying causes and implementing preventive measures, such as providing sufficient space, environmental enrichment, balanced nutrition, and appropriate flock management, these behaviors can be minimized or corrected. Regular monitoring, behavioral modifications, and seeking professional advice when necessary are essential for maintaining a harmonious and healthy flock. Remember, a proactive and holistic approach is key to promoting the overall well-being of your chickens.

Nutritional Disorders

Proper nutrition plays a vital role in the overall health and well-being of chickens. Just like humans, chickens can also suffer from various nutritional disorders that can have detrimental effects on their health. In this article, we will delve into three common nutritional disorders: obesity, excess calcium, and vitamin/mineral deficiencies. We will specifically discuss these disorders in the context of the Chicken Health Bible, aiming to provide comprehensive insights for poultry enthusiasts and farmers.

Obesity in Chickens:

Obesity is a prevalent nutritional disorder among chickens that results from an imbalance between energy intake and expenditure. Chickens with access to high-calorie feeds and limited physical activity are particularly susceptible to obesity. The Chicken Health Bible emphasizes the importance of maintaining a healthy weight in chickens to prevent a range of associated health issues, including cardiovascular problems, joint disorders, and reduced egg production. Proper diet management and encouraging exercise are crucial for preventing and managing obesity in chickens.

Excess Calcium:

Calcium is an essential mineral required for strong bones, eggshell production, and muscle function in chickens. However, excessive calcium intake can lead to a condition known as hypercalcemia. The Chicken Health Bible educates poultry keepers about the risks of providing excessive calcium supplements or feeds rich in calcium. Hypercalcemia can cause kidney damage, reduced eggshell quality, and impaired growth. By following recommended calcium supplementation guidelines, poultry enthusiasts can prevent these issues and ensure optimal calcium levels for their chickens.

Vitamin and Mineral Deficiencies:

Chickens require a balanced intake of vitamins and minerals for proper growth, immune function, and overall health. Deficiencies in essential nutrients such as vitamins A, D, E, B-complex, and minerals like iron, zinc, and selenium can lead to a range of disorders. The Chicken Health Bible advises poultry keepers on the importance of providing a varied and nutritionally complete diet to their chickens. It highlights the symptoms associated with specific deficiencies, such as poor feather quality, reduced egg production, skeletal abnormalities, and increased susceptibility to infections. By identifying and addressing these deficiencies, chicken owners can optimize the health and productivity of their flocks.

Nutritional disorders, including obesity, excess calcium, and vitamin/mineral deficiencies, can significantly impact the health and productivity of chickens. The Chicken Health Bible serves as a valuable resource, offering guidance to poultry enthusiasts on how to prevent, identify, and manage these disorders. By understanding the importance of a balanced diet, appropriate supplementation, and regular exercise, chicken owners can ensure their flocks thrive and lead healthy lives. Remember, a well-nourished chicken is a happy and productive chicken.

How to Recognize Sources of Poisonings in Your Backyard

Creating a safe and healthy environment for your backyard chickens is crucial for their well-being. While you may have taken necessary measures to protect your flock, there are potential sources of poisonings that can go unnoticed. In this guide, we will explore various sources of poisonings that can affect backyard chickens and discuss how to recognize and prevent them. Specifically, we will focus on botulism, household poisons, lead poisoning, mold toxins in feed (mycotoxins), toxic gas, toxic foods, and plants. By understanding these risks, you can ensure the health and safety of your feathered friends.

Botulism:

Botulism is a serious condition caused by the toxin produced by the bacterium Clostridium botulinum. Chickens can contract botulism by ingesting contaminated food, water, or carcasses. Common signs of botulism in chickens include difficulty breathing, paralysis, weakness, and drooping wings. To recognize and prevent botulism, ensure proper sanitation practices, eliminate potential sources of contamination, and provide clean and fresh food and water.

Household Poisons:

Various household poisons pose a significant risk to chickens. Common substances such as cleaning products, pesticides, herbicides, and rodenticides can be toxic if ingested. Symptoms of poisoning may vary depending on the specific substance but can include lethargy, difficulty breathing, seizures, and gastrointestinal issues. Store chemicals securely, use them cautiously, and keep chickens away from treated areas to prevent accidental poisonings.

Lead Poisoning:

Lead poisoning can occur when chickens ingest lead-containing substances such as peeling paint, lead-based objects, or contaminated soil. Lead affects the nervous system and can lead to neurological problems, weakness, weight loss, and even death. To prevent lead poisoning, avoid exposing chickens to lead-containing materials, ensure access to uncontaminated soil, and consider lead testing if you suspect a potential source.

Mold Toxins in Feed (Mycotoxins):

Mycotoxins are toxic compounds produced by certain molds that can contaminate poultry feed.

Consuming feed contaminated with mycotoxins can lead to various health issues, including reduced growth, immune system suppression, organ damage, and even death. Signs of mycotoxin poisoning may include decreased feed intake, poor performance, and abnormalities in egg production. To minimize the risk, store feed in cool and dry conditions, regularly inspect for mold growth, and consider mycotoxin testing for feed sources.

Toxic Gas:

Poor ventilation in chicken coops can result in the accumulation of toxic gases, such as ammonia and carbon monoxide. Exposure to these gases can cause respiratory distress, eye irritation, decreased egg production, and even death. Ensure proper airflow and ventilation in the coop to prevent toxic gas buildup and maintain good respiratory health for your chickens.

Toxic Foods and Plants:

Certain foods and plants can be toxic to chickens and should be avoided. Examples include avocado, chocolate, caffeine, onions, nightshade plants, and many others. Symptoms of food or plant poisoning in chickens may include weakness, diarrhea, tremors, and reduced egg production. Familiarize yourself with the list of toxic foods and plants and ensure your chickens' access to a safe and well-balanced diet.

Maintaining a safe backyard environment for your chickens is essential for their overall health and well-being. By being aware of potential sources of poisonings such as botulism, household poisons, lead poisoning, mycotoxins, toxic gases, toxic foods, and plants, you can take preventive measures to protect your flock. Regularly inspect the surroundings, provide clean and uncontaminated resources, and seek veterinary assistance promptly if you suspect any poisoning-related symptoms in your chickens. With proper knowledge and vigilance, you can ensure a happy and healthy environment for your feathered companions.

How to Identify Housing and Environmental Dangers

Creating a safe and healthy environment for chickens is crucial for their overall well-being and productivity. As responsible chicken keepers, it is important to be aware of potential housing and environmental dangers that can negatively impact the health of our feathered friends. This comprehensive guide will focus on five specific dangers: frostbite, hardware disease, heat stress, starve-outs, and suffocation. By understanding and identifying these risks, we can take appropriate measures to prevent them and ensure the optimal health of our chickens.

Frostbite: Hardware Disease:

Frostbite occurs when a chicken's tissues freeze due to prolonged exposure to extremely cold temperatures. It commonly affects the comb, wattles, and toes. To identify frostbite, look for signs such as pale, discolored, or blackened skin, swelling, or the presence of blisters. To prevent frostbite, provide adequate shelter with insulation, ventilation, and drafts-free areas. Applying petroleum jelly or other protective ointments to vulnerable areas can also help.

Hardware disease refers to the ingestion of foreign objects by chickens, which can lead to injuries or infections. Chickens often peck at small metal or sharp objects, mistaking them for food. To identify hardware disease, watch for symptoms like loss of appetite, reduced egg production, droopy appearance, and diarrhea. To prevent it, regularly inspect the coop and surrounding areas for potential hazards and provide a clean and clutter-free environment.

Heat Stress:

Heat stress occurs when chickens are exposed to high temperatures and struggle to regulate their body temperature effectively. This can lead to dehydration, reduced egg production, and even death. Signs of heat stress include panting, drooping wings, reduced activity, and disinterest in food. To prevent heat stress, ensure proper ventilation, provide shade, offer cool water, and consider using misters or fans during hot weather.

Starve-outs:

Starve-outs, also known as starvation or malnutrition, happen when chickens do not receive adequate nutrition. This can occur due to poor feeding practices, competition for food, or inadequate access to water and feed. Signs of starve-outs include weight loss, decreased activity, weakness, poor feather quality, and reduced egg production. To prevent this, ensure a balanced diet with appropriate nutrition, provide sufficient feeders and waterers, and monitor the flock's feeding habits regularly.

Suffocation:

Suffocation is a severe danger in chicken coops, particularly for chicks or small birds. It can occur when chickens overcrowd or get trapped in small spaces, leading to inadequate airflow. Signs of suffocation include gasping for air, panic, and agitation. To prevent suffocation, maintain proper spacing between chickens, avoid overcrowding, and ensure the coop has adequate ventilation. Regularly inspect the coop for potential hazards that could lead to entrapment.

Maintaining a safe and healthy environment for chickens is essential for their overall well-being. By being aware of housing and environmental dangers such as frostbite, hardware disease, heat stress, starve-outs, and suffocation, chicken keepers can take proactive measures to prevent these risks. Regularly monitoring the flock, providing appropriate shelter, ensuring a balanced diet, and practicing good husbandry techniques will go a long way in safeguarding the health and vitality of your chickens. Remember, a healthy flock is a happy flock!

Chapter 15

Diagnostic Guides

Welcome to Chapter 15 of the Chicken Health Bible! In this chapter, we will delve into the important topic of diagnostic guides for chicken health. Keeping a flock of healthy chickens requires not only proactive care but also the ability to identify and address potential health issues promptly. Diagnostic guides are invaluable tools that enable poultry owners to recognize symptoms, make accurate diagnoses, and provide appropriate treatment for their feathered friends.

In this chapter, we will explore various aspects of diagnostic guides and their significance in maintaining the well-being of your flock. We will discuss the importance of observation skills and how to develop a keen eye for detecting signs of illness or distress in chickens. By learning to identify abnormal behaviors, physical changes, and other indicators, you will be better equipped to assess the overall health of your birds.

Additionally, this chapter will cover different diagnostic techniques that can aid in determining the root cause of chicken health problems. We will delve into the use of physical examination, laboratory tests, and other diagnostic tools commonly employed by poultry veterinarians. Understanding these techniques will empower you to collaborate effectively with professionals or even conduct basic assessments on your own, when appropriate.

Furthermore, we will explore specific diagnostic guides for common poultry ailments and diseases. From respiratory infections to parasitic infestations, this chapter will provide comprehensive information on how to recognize and diagnose these conditions. By familiarizing yourself with the characteristic symptoms, you will be able to intervene early, potentially preventing the spread of disease and minimizing its impact on your flock.

Finally, we will discuss the significance of record-keeping and documenting observations when it comes to diagnostic guides. By maintaining detailed records of your flock's health, behavior, and any treatments administered, you can establish valuable patterns and trends. These records can serve as a valuable reference for future diagnoses, enabling you to make informed decisions and track the effectiveness of various interventions.

As you progress through this chapter, you will gain a deeper understanding of diagnostic guides and their role in promoting the well-being of your chickens. By becoming adept at recognizing signs of illness, employing diagnostic techniques, and maintaining accurate records, you will be better equipped to address health concerns and maintain a healthy and thriving flock.

So let us dive into the world of diagnostic guides and equip ourselves with the knowledge to ensure the continued health and happiness of our feathered companions!

Getting Advice or Going It Alone

Keeping a healthy and thriving flock of chickens requires knowledge, experience, and sometimes, professional guidance. As a chicken keeper, you may find yourself faced with various challenges and questions regarding the health and well-being of your feathered friends. In such situations, you might wonder whether to seek advice from professionals or rely solely on your own judgment and resources. This article aims to explore the benefits of both options and provide insights into finding professionals who can assist you in ensuring the optimal health of your flock, specifically within the context of the Chicken Health Bible.

When it comes to maintaining the well-being of your chickens, there are certain instances where seeking professional advice becomes crucial. These situations may include:

1. **Disease Diagnosis and Treatment:** If you notice any unusual symptoms or behavior in your chickens, consulting a veterinarian or an experienced poultry health specialist can be immensely beneficial. They possess the knowledge and expertise to diagnose and treat various diseases that may affect your flock.
2. **Preventive Measures:** Professionals can guide you on implementing preventive measures to safeguard your flock against common diseases and parasites. They can provide valuable insights on vaccination schedules, biosecurity practices, and proper sanitation measures to minimize the risk of infections.
3. **Nutritional Guidance:** A well-balanced diet is essential for the overall health and productivity of your chickens. Professionals can offer advice on formulating appropriate feed and supplement plans based on the specific needs of your flock, taking into consideration factors such as age, breed, and purpose (e.g., egg-laying or meat production).
4. **Breeding and Genetics:** If you are interested in breeding your chickens or improving specific traits within your flock, professionals can provide expertise in areas such as genetic selection, breeding techniques, and hatchery management. This guidance can help you achieve your desired breeding goals effectively.

While seeking professional help is valuable, it is also important to develop your own knowledge and skills as a chicken keeper. Going it alone can empower you to become more self-reliant and make informed decisions based on your understanding of your flock's specific needs. Here are some reasons why you might choose to rely on your own resources:

1. **Empowerment and Independence:** By acquiring knowledge through resources like the Chicken Health Bible and other reliable references, you can develop a deeper understanding of chicken health and welfare. This empowers you to make educated decisions independently, thus fostering a sense of accomplishment and self-sufficiency.
2. **Immediate Action:** In some cases, you may not have immediate access to professional assistance. By relying on your own knowledge and experience, you can quickly assess and address minor health issues or emergencies that may arise within your flock, potentially saving valuable time and minimizing risks.
3. **Cost-Effectiveness:** Consulting professionals regularly can be expensive, especially for small-scale chicken keepers. By building your expertise and implementing preventive measures, you can reduce the need for frequent professional assistance, thereby saving costs while still maintaining a healthy flock.

To strike a balance between seeking professional guidance and going it alone, consider the following strategies for finding professionals who can assist you:

1. **Local Veterinarians:** Reach out to local veterinarians who specialize in poultry or farm animals. They can provide expert advice, diagnose illnesses, and offer treatment options tailored to your flock's specific needs.
2. **Poultry Extension Services:** Many agricultural universities or cooperative extension offices have poultry experts who offer guidance and support to farmers and backyard chicken keepers. They often provide resources, workshops, and access to diagnostic laboratories for disease testing.
3. **Poultry Associations and Clubs:** Joining local or national poultry associations and clubs can connect you with experienced chicken keepers and professionals in the field. These organizations often organize workshops, seminars, and conferences where you can learn from experts and network with like-minded individuals.
4. **Online Communities and Forums:** Participating in online forums and communities dedicated to poultry keeping can provide you with a wealth of knowledge and the opportunity to seek advice from experienced chicken keepers and professionals worldwide. However, exercise caution and verify information from reliable sources.

When it comes to the health and well-being of your flock, striking a balance between seeking professional guidance and relying on your own resources is essential. By leveraging professional expertise and developing your own knowledge, you can create an environment where your chickens thrive. The Chicken Health Bible and other resources can serve as valuable references, while local veterinarians, poultry extension services, associations, and online communities can connect you with professionals who can assist you on your chicken-keeping journey. Remember, a healthy flock is a happy flock, and by investing in their well-being, you are ensuring the longevity and productivity of your feathery companions.

How to Collect Samples for Your Chicken-Health Advisor

Maintaining the health of your chickens is crucial for their overall well-being and productivity. To effectively diagnose and address health issues, it is essential to collect accurate and representative samples for analysis by a chicken health advisor. This guide aims to provide detailed instructions on how to collect samples for various purposes, including submitting a chicken for postmortem examination and collecting specimens for parasite identification. By following these guidelines, you can ensure that your chickens receive the best possible care and treatment.

Submitting a Chicken for Postmortem Examination, also known as necropsy, is a valuable tool for diagnosing the cause of a chicken's death and identifying potential health concerns within your flock. Here's a step-by-step guide on how to collect and submit a chicken for postmortem examination:

1. **Choose the right candidate:** Select a recently deceased bird that best represents the symptoms or issues observed in your flock.
2. **Handle the bird with care:** Wear disposable gloves and avoid unnecessary contact with the carcass to minimize contamination and preserve the condition of the specimen.
3. **Store and transport the carcass:** Place the chicken in a clean, leak-proof plastic bag or wrap it in a plastic sheet to prevent any fluids from leaking. Keep the carcass cool during transportation, but avoid freezing it.
4. **Document relevant information:** Before submitting the bird, note down any pertinent details such as the bird's breed, age, symptoms, and recent changes in behavior or diet.
5. **Contact a chicken health advisor or veterinarian:** Reach out to a reputable chicken health advisor or veterinarian who can guide you through the process of submitting the carcass for postmortem examination. Follow their instructions regarding packaging, shipping, and the necessary forms or paperwork.

Collecting Specimens for Parasite Identification Parasites can significantly impact the health and productivity of your chickens. Collecting appropriate specimens for parasite identification is vital for accurate diagnosis and treatment. Here's a step-by-step guide on how to collect samples for parasite identification:

1. **Determine the type of specimen required:** Parasite identification may involve collecting feces, feathers, skin scrapings, blood samples, or other relevant specimens. Consult with your chicken health advisor or veterinarian to identify the specific samples needed.
2. **Prepare the collection materials:** Gather clean, sterile containers or collection kits suitable for the specimen type. Label each container with the bird's identification and the date of collection.
3. **Fecal sample collection:** To collect a fecal sample, place a clean plastic bag or container beneath the chicken and gently massage the lower abdomen to encourage defecation. Collect a small amount of fresh feces, preferably without any bedding material, and seal the container tightly.
4. **Feather and skin scrapings:** If mites or other external parasites are suspected, use a clean,

fine-toothed comb or a scalpel to collect feathers and scrape the skin gently. Collect samples from several birds if possible, to ensure accuracy.
5. **Blood sample collection:** Collecting blood samples for parasite identification usually requires veterinary assistance. Consult with a veterinarian experienced in poultry health to guide you through the process.
6. **Packaging and transportation:** Securely seal each specimen container, ensuring no leakage or cross-contamination. Keep the samples cool, but avoid freezing, during transportation to the laboratory or clinic.
7. **Provide relevant information:** Along with the specimens, include information about the flock's symptoms, treatment history, and any other relevant details. This additional information will assist the chicken health advisor or veterinarian in making an accurate diagnosis.

Collecting samples for your chicken health advisor is a crucial step in diagnosing and addressing health issues in your flock. By following the guidelines provided in this comprehensive guide, you can ensure that the samples you collect are representative, well-preserved, and accurately identified by the appropriate professionals. Remember, early detection and proper treatment are key to maintaining the health and well-being of your chickens.

How to Perform a DIY Postmortem

Performing a postmortem examination, also known as a necropsy, on a chicken can provide valuable insights into its health and help diagnose potential issues that may have led to its death. Conducting a DIY postmortem allows chicken owners to gain a better understanding of the overall flock's health and make informed decisions to prevent future illnesses. In this article, we will guide you through the process of gathering equipment, getting started, and performing a necropsy on a chicken.

Gathering Equipment:

Before starting the postmortem, it's crucial to assemble the necessary equipment to ensure a smooth and efficient examination. Here are the essential tools you will need:

1. **Personal Protective Equipment (PPE):** Wear gloves, goggles, and a lab coat or apron to protect yourself from any potential pathogens.
2. **Necropsy Kit:** Purchase or create a necropsy kit that includes sharp dissection scissors, a scalpel or razor blade, blunt-nosed forceps, a bone saw, and a cutting board.
3. **Disposable Bags:** Prepare several plastic bags to contain different organs or tissues during the examination.
4. **Labels and Marker:** Use labels and a marker to identify each sample or organ to prevent confusion later on.

Getting Started:

Once you have all the necessary equipment, follow these steps to perform a DIY postmortem on a chicken:

1. **Choose the Appropriate Setting:** Find a clean, well-lit area to conduct the necropsy. It could be a dedicated workspace, or a clean table covered with disposable materials.
2. **Prepare the Chicken:** If the chicken has recently passed away, refrigerate it to slow down decomposition. Ensure the chicken is completely thawed if it had been previously frozen.
3. **External Examination:** Begin by examining the chicken externally. Note any abnormalities, such as skin lesions, feather loss, or signs of trauma.
4. **Open the Body Cavity:** Using the scalpel or razor blade, make an incision from the keel bone (breastbone) down towards the vent. Be cautious not to puncture any underlying organs.
5. **Observe the Organs:** Upon opening the body cavity, examine the organs for any signs of abnormalities, discoloration, or inflammation. Pay close attention to the liver, spleen, heart, lungs, kidneys, and intestines.
6. **Collect Samples:** If you notice any suspicious lesions or abnormalities, collect samples of affected tissues for further examination. Use the dissection scissors and forceps to carefully remove tissues, placing each sample in a labeled bag.
7. **Document Findings:** Take detailed notes or photographs of any abnormalities observed during the necropsy. This documentation will be helpful when seeking advice or discussing the findings with a veterinarian.

Necropsy of a Chicken:

Now, let's focus specifically on the necropsy procedure for a chicken:

1. **Identify Cause of Death:** The primary objective of a necropsy is to determine the cause of death. Look for signs of disease, such as changes in the organs, lesions, or evidence of parasites.
2. **Examine the Respiratory System:** Check the trachea, lungs, and air sacs for any signs of respiratory diseases, such as congestion, excess mucus, or abnormal tissue.
3. **Inspect the Digestive System:** Evaluate the crop, proventriculus (glandular stomach), gizzard, intestines, and ceca for any abnormalities, such as inflammation, ulcers, or blockages.
4. **Evaluate the Liver:** The liver plays a vital role in overall health. Look for signs of disease, discoloration, or enlargement.
5. **Assess the Heart and Blood Vessels:** Examine the heart and major blood vessels for abnormalities, including evidence of infection, clots, or structural issues.
6. **Examine the Reproductive Organs:** In the case of hens, evaluate the oviduct, ovaries, and shell gland for abnormalities or signs of infection. For roosters, inspect the testes and associated structures.

Performing a DIY postmortem or necropsy on a chicken can provide valuable insights into the health and causes of death within a flock. By following the steps outlined in this guide, chicken owners can gain a better understanding of their flock's overall health, detect potential diseases or infections, and make informed decisions to maintain the well-being of their chickens. Remember, if you encounter any uncertainties or complex findings, consult a veterinarian for further guidance.

Chapter 16

Medicating And Vaccinating Backyard Flocks

Welcome to Chapter 16 of the Chicken Health Bible, where we delve into the crucial topic of medicating and vaccinating backyard flocks. As proud chicken keepers, we understand the importance of maintaining the health and well-being of our feathered friends. Just like any living creature, chickens can be susceptible to various diseases and infections that can impact their overall health and productivity. To ensure the longevity and vitality of our backyard flocks, it is essential to be knowledgeable about medicating and vaccinating practices.

In this chapter, we will explore the fundamentals of medicating and vaccinating backyard flocks, providing you with the necessary information and guidance to make informed decisions for the health of your chickens. We will cover a range of topics, including the types of medications and vaccines available, their uses, administration methods, and important considerations to keep in mind.

Understanding the various diseases that can affect chickens is the first step in protecting your flock. We will discuss common poultry diseases, such as Newcastle disease, Marek's disease, coccidiosis, infectious bronchitis, and many others. You will learn how to identify the symptoms, prevent the spread of diseases, and implement effective treatment strategies.

Medication plays a crucial role in managing and treating diseases in chickens. We will explore different types of medications, including antibiotics, antiparasitics, and antifungals, along with their applications and potential side effects. Understanding proper dosage, administration methods, and withdrawal periods is vital for ensuring the safety of both your chickens and the consumers of their products.

Vaccination is a powerful tool in preventing the onset and spread of diseases within your flock. We will guide you through the process of selecting appropriate vaccines, understanding vaccination schedules, and proper administration techniques. By incorporating a well-planned vaccination program, you can significantly reduce the risk of disease outbreaks and provide your chickens with a stronger immune system.

Additionally, we will address other aspects related to medicating and vaccinating backyard flocks, such as biosecurity measures, record-keeping, and consulting with veterinary professionals. Proper biosecurity practices can help minimize the introduction and spread of diseases, safeguarding the health of your flock. Keeping detailed records of medications, vaccinations, and any observed symptoms will prove invaluable in maintaining a healthy and productive flock. Consulting with veterinarians and poultry experts can provide you with expert guidance and support when dealing with challenging health issues.

By the end of this chapter, you will have gained comprehensive knowledge about medicating and vaccinating backyard flocks. Armed with this information, you will be better equipped to protect your chickens from diseases and ensure their optimal health and welfare.

Remember, a healthy flock is a happy flock, and we are here to empower you to become a skilled caretaker for your beloved backyard chickens. So, let's embark on this important journey together and become guardians of our flock's well-being.

The Link between Drugs and Food-Producing Animals:

As food-producing animals, chickens are subject to regulations and guidelines to ensure the safety of the food they provide. The use of medications, including antibiotics, in poultry farming raises concerns about the potential impact on human health. Antibiotics used in livestock can contribute to the development of antibiotic-resistant bacteria, which pose a significant public health threat.

Regulations and Guidelines:

In many countries, including the United States, regulatory agencies such as the Food and Drug Administration (FDA) and the United States Department of Agriculture (USDA) closely monitor the use of antibiotics in food-producing animals. They set guidelines and enforce regulations to promote responsible use and minimize the risk of antibiotic resistance. These regulations often dictate the types of antibiotics approved for use in chickens, withdrawal periods before slaughter, and proper dosages.

Responsible Antibiotic Use:

Responsible antibiotic use in backyard flocks is crucial to safeguard both the chickens' health and the health of consumers. Here are some key considerations:

1. **Veterinary Guidance**: Always consult a veterinarian before administering antibiotics to your chickens. A professional can provide appropriate diagnoses, treatment plans, and guidance on dosage and duration of treatment.
2. **Proper Diagnosis:** Accurate diagnosis is essential to identify the specific bacteria causing the infection. This helps determine the most effective antibiotic and ensures targeted treatment.

3. **Follow Dosage Instructions:** Adhere strictly to the recommended dosage instructions provided by the veterinarian. Overdosing or underdosing can lead to ineffective treatment or antibiotic resistance.
4. **Withdrawal Periods:** Respect the withdrawal periods recommended by regulatory agencies. These periods ensure that antibiotics are no longer present in the chickens' system at the time of slaughter, minimizing the risk of antibiotic residues in meat and eggs.
5. **Record Keeping:** Maintain detailed records of the medications administered to individual chickens, including the type, dosage, and duration of treatment. This information is valuable for future reference and can assist veterinarians in making informed decisions.

Vaccination:

In addition to antibiotics, vaccines play a crucial role in preventing and controlling diseases in backyard flocks. Vaccination helps build immunity against common poultry diseases, reducing the need for antibiotic use. It is important to note that vaccines are not a substitute for good husbandry practices and biosecurity measures. Here are some key points on vaccination:

1. **Disease Identification:** Work with a veterinarian to identify the prevalent diseases in your region and determine the appropriate vaccines for your flock. Different areas may have varying disease risks, so tailored vaccination protocols are necessary.
2. **Proper Storage and Handling:** Vaccines are sensitive to temperature and handling. Follow the manufacturer's instructions for proper storage and administration to ensure vaccine effectiveness.
3. **Vaccination Schedule:** Develop a vaccination schedule based on the age and health status of your flock. Some vaccines require multiple doses or booster shots, while others are administered only once.
4. **Documentation:** Keep accurate records of the vaccines administered, including the vaccine type, date, and batch number. These records are essential for tracking the flock's vaccination status and providing information to veterinarians or buyers if necessary.

Medicating and vaccinating backyard flocks is an integral part of responsible chicken ownership. When it comes to antibiotics, following veterinary guidance, using proper dosages, respecting withdrawal periods, and keeping records are vital. Vaccination, coupled with good husbandry practices and biosecurity measures, helps prevent diseases and reduces the need for antibiotics. By implementing these practices, backyard flock owners can ensure the health and well-being of their chickens while minimizing the potential risks to human health.

To Vaccinate or Not to Vaccinate? Pros and Cons

In recent years, backyard chicken farming has gained popularity among urban and rural dwellers alike. While it offers numerous benefits, such as fresh eggs and the joy of raising animals, it also comes with its own set of challenges, including the need to prioritize chicken health. One crucial aspect of chicken health management is vaccination. This article explores the pros and cons of vaccinating backyard chickens and provides insights into successfully vaccinating your flock.

Pros of Vaccinating Backyard Chickens:

1. **Disease Prevention:** Vaccines are designed to protect chickens from harmful pathogens that can cause severe diseases. By vaccinating your flock, you reduce the risk of outbreaks and help maintain the overall health and well-being of your chickens.
2. **Improved Immune Response:** Vaccines stimulate the chicken's immune system, enabling it to recognize and fight specific diseases. This leads to a stronger immune response and increases the chances of chickens effectively combating infections if exposed.
3. **Reduced Mortality:** Vaccines play a crucial role in reducing chicken mortality rates by preventing or minimizing the severity of diseases. Vaccinated chickens are more likely to survive and thrive, ensuring a healthier and more productive flock.
4. **Cost-Effective:** Investing in vaccines is often more cost-effective than treating diseases or replacing chickens lost to illness. Vaccinations help minimize veterinary expenses and potential losses in egg production, resulting in long-term financial savings.

Cons of Vaccinating Backyard Chickens:

1. **Risk of Vaccine Side Effects:** While rare, there is a small possibility of adverse reactions to vaccines, including swelling at the injection site or mild illness. However, these side effects are generally temporary and mild compared to the potential consequences of contracting the actual diseases.
2. **Limited Availability:** Some vaccines may not be readily available for backyard chicken owners. Certain vaccines might be designed and distributed primarily for commercial poultry operations, making it challenging to access specific vaccines for individual backyard flocks.
3. **Difficulty in Administration:** Administering vaccines can be a challenging task for inexperienced chicken owners. It requires proper handling, storage, and precise administration techniques. Without appropriate knowledge and training, there is a risk of improper vaccination, which could lead to ineffective protection.

Vaccinating Successfully:

1. **Consult with a Poultry Veterinarian:** Seek guidance from a poultry veterinarian who can provide valuable advice on the vaccines suitable for your flock's specific needs. They can help you design an appropriate vaccination schedule and ensure correct administration.
2. **Educate Yourself:** Learn about the common diseases affecting chickens in your region and understand the benefits and risks associated with relevant vaccines. Reliable sources, such as reputable poultry publications or university extension services, can provide accurate information to help you make informed decisions.
3. **Follow Best Practices:** Handle vaccines according to the manufacturer's instructions, ensuring proper storage conditions and maintaining the cold chain if required. Use sterile

equipment for administration and maintain proper hygiene to prevent contamination during vaccination.
4. **Maintain Records:** Keep detailed records of the vaccines administered, including the brand, batch number, date of administration, and the individual chickens vaccinated. This information will be crucial for future reference, tracking vaccine efficacy, and complying with any regulatory requirements.

Vaccinating backyard chickens is a crucial aspect of maintaining their health and preventing diseases. While there are potential risks and challenges associated with vaccination, the benefits of disease prevention, improved immune response, and reduced mortality outweigh the cons. By consulting with experts, educating yourself, and following best practices, you can successfully vaccinate your flock and ensure a healthier and happier backyard chicken experience.

Medications and Vaccinations

Maintaining the health of chickens is crucial for poultry farmers and backyard chicken enthusiasts alike. Along with proper nutrition, hygiene, and regular veterinary care, medications and vaccinations play a vital role in safeguarding the well-being of these birds. In this comprehensive guide, we will explore different administration methods for medications and vaccines, including drinking water, oral administration, eyedrops, wing web stab, subcutaneous injection, and intramuscular injection. Understanding these techniques will empower chicken owners to make informed decisions regarding their flock's health and ensure optimal disease prevention and treatment.

Medications and Vaccinations in Drinking Water:

Importance and Application:

- Administering medications and vaccines through drinking water is a practical method to treat or vaccinate a large number of chickens simultaneously.
- It is commonly used for medications such as antibiotics, coccidiostats, and anticoccidials.

Procedure:

- Follow the dosage instructions provided by the medication or vaccine manufacturer.
- Calculate the appropriate amount of medication or vaccine based on the water volume and the number of birds.
- Mix the medication or vaccine thoroughly in clean, fresh water.
- Ensure that the medicated water is the sole water source available to the chickens during the specified treatment period.

Medications and Vaccinations by Mouth:

Importance and Application:

- Oral administration is often used for medications that need to be directly ingested by

chickens.
- It allows targeted treatment for specific ailments, such as deworming or vitamin deficiencies.

Procedure:
- Administer the medication using a syringe or dropper.
- Gently open the chicken's beak and carefully deliver the medication towards the back of the throat.
- Ensure the chicken swallows the medication, avoiding aspiration into the respiratory system.

Medications and Vaccinations via Eyedrop:

Importance and Application:
- Eyedrops are used to treat eye infections or administer specific eye-related medications.
- They can also be used to deliver vaccines against certain diseases.

Procedure:
- Gently restrain the chicken and keep its head steady.
- Administer the prescribed number of drops directly onto the eye surface, avoiding contact with the dropper tip.

Medications and Vaccinations through Wing Web Stab:

Importance and Application:
- Wing web stab method is employed for vaccination against certain diseases, such as Marek's disease.
- It allows for easy and effective vaccine administration, stimulating immunity.

Procedure:
- Restrain the chicken and expose the wing web area, which is the thin, translucent skin between the primary and secondary feathers.
- Make a small puncture in the wing web using a sterile needle or lancet.
- Apply a drop of the vaccine onto the puncture site and ensure proper absorption.

Medications and Vaccinations Under the Skin (Subcutaneous Injection):

Importance and Application:
- Subcutaneous injections are commonly used for administering vaccines, antibiotics, or other medications that require a more controlled delivery method.
- This technique allows for accurate dosing and efficient absorption.

Procedure:
- Restrain the chicken securely, ensuring a stable and calm environment.
- Select an appropriate injection site, typically the loose skin on the back of the neck.
- Use a sterile syringe and needle to deliver the medication or vaccine just beneath the skin.
- Dispose of used needles and syringes safely.

Medications and Vaccinations in the Muscle (Intramuscular Injection):

Importance and Application:
- Intramuscular injections are used for certain medications or vaccines that require direct administration into the muscle tissue.
- This method ensures rapid absorption and distribution throughout the body.

Procedure:
- Restrain the chicken securely to minimize movement.
- Identify the appropriate injection site, usually the breast or thigh muscle.
- Use a sterile syringe and needle to inject the medication or vaccine deep into the muscle tissue.
- Dispose of used needles and syringes properly.

Medications and vaccinations are essential components of maintaining chicken health. Understanding the various administration methods, including drinking water, oral administration, eyedrops, wing web stab, subcutaneous injection, and intramuscular injection, empowers chicken owners to proactively address health concerns and prevent diseases. Remember, it is crucial to consult with a veterinarian for proper diagnosis, treatment, and vaccination protocols specific to your flock's needs. By following best practices and utilizing appropriate techniques, you can enhance the overall health and well-being of your chickens and ensure their productive and fulfilling lives.

Chapter 17

Chicken First Aid

Welcome to Chapter 17 of the Chicken Health Bible, where we will delve into the essential topic of Chicken First Aid. As chicken keepers, it is crucial to be well-prepared to handle any health emergencies that may arise within your flock. Prompt and appropriate action during times of distress can make a significant difference in the well-being and survival of your chickens. In this chapter, we will cover the fundamentals of chicken first aid, including common injuries and illnesses, emergency care, and preventive measures.

Assessing the Situation:

When encountering an injured or sick chicken, the first step is to assess the situation calmly and quickly. Observe the bird's behavior, breathing, appetite, and general appearance. Isolate the affected chicken from the rest of the flock to prevent the spread of any potential infections. Remember, handling an injured or distressed chicken can be stressful for both you and the bird, so approach with care and confidence.

Basic First Aid Supplies:

Having a well-stocked first aid kit specifically designed for chicken care is essential. Here are some basic supplies to include:

a) Disposable gloves
b) Sterile gauze pads and bandages
c) Antiseptic solution or wipes
d) Scissors
e) Tweezers
f) Sterile saline solution for flushing wounds
g) Styptic powder to stop bleeding

h) Heat source (such as a heating pad or warm water bottle)

Common Injuries and Illnesses:

Understanding the signs and symptoms of common chicken injuries and illnesses can help you provide the appropriate first aid. Some typical issues include:

1. **Wounds:** Cuts, scrapes, and punctures can occur due to predator attacks or aggressive behavior among flock members. Clean wounds with an antiseptic solution, apply pressure to stop bleeding, and bandage if necessary.
2. **Respiratory Issues:** Symptoms include sneezing, coughing, wheezing, and nasal discharge. Isolate the affected bird and provide a warm, clean, and well-ventilated environment. Consult a veterinarian if the condition worsens.
3. **Bumblefoot:** This condition manifests as a swollen and infected foot pad. Soak the foot in warm water with Epsom salts, gently clean the area, and apply antibiotic ointment. Bandage the foot to prevent further injury.
4. **Crop Issues:** A sour or impacted crop can lead to digestive problems. Massage the crop gently, provide plenty of fresh water, and feed a soft or liquid diet until the crop empties. Seek veterinary advice if the issue persists.
5. **Egg Binding:** When a hen is unable to pass an egg, it can become a life-threatening condition. Soak the hen in warm water to help relax the muscles, apply a lubricant, and gently massage the abdomen. If unsuccessful, seek immediate veterinary assistance.

Emergency Care:

Certain situations require immediate attention and may not allow time for veterinary intervention. Here are some emergency measures to take:

1. **Bleeding:** Apply direct pressure to the wound using a clean cloth or gauze pad. Elevate the affected area if possible and use styptic powder or cornstarch to aid in clotting.
2. **Shock:** Keep the bird warm and quiet, away from drafts and noise. Offer electrolytes and glucose in their drinking water to help stabilize their condition.
3. **Heatstroke:** Move the chicken to a cool and shaded area. Provide fresh water and gently wet the bird's feathers with cool (not cold) water. Monitor their temperature and behavior closely.
4. **Poisoning:** Remove the chicken from the source of poisoning and contact a veterinarian immediately. Provide activated charcoal if advised.

Preventive Measures:

Preventing injuries and illnesses is crucial for maintaining the overall health of your flock. Implement the following preventive measures:

1. Maintain a clean and well-ventilated coop.
2. Regularly inspect the flock for signs of illness or injury.

3. Provide a balanced diet and clean water.
4. Minimize stress by ensuring sufficient space and social interactions.
5. Quarantine new birds before introducing them to the flock.
6. Conduct regular parasite control.

Being equipped with the knowledge and supplies for chicken first aid is an essential aspect of responsible chicken keeping. By promptly recognizing and addressing injuries and illnesses, you can improve the chances of a positive outcome for your flock. However, always remember that professional veterinary care should be sought for severe or persistent conditions. Stay vigilant, stay prepared, and prioritize the health and well-being of your feathered friends.

Remember, a healthy flock is a happy flock!

Chapter 18

Your Chickens And Your Health

In the previous chapters of the Chicken Health Bible, we discussed various aspects of raising healthy chickens, including nutrition, housing, and disease prevention. However, it is essential not only to consider the well-being of your feathered friends but also to understand the potential impact of chicken health on your own well-being. In Chapter 18, we will explore the intricate relationship between your chickens and your health, highlighting both the benefits and potential risks associated with poultry ownership.

Physical Health Benefits:

Keeping chickens can offer numerous physical health benefits for poultry owners. Here are some ways that interacting with chickens can positively impact your well-being:

1. **Fresh and Nutritious Eggs**: Raising your own chickens allows you to have a regular supply of fresh eggs, which are a rich source of essential nutrients. Eggs are known to be a good source of protein, vitamins, and minerals, contributing to a well-balanced diet.
2. **Physical Activity:** Taking care of chickens involves various physical activities like feeding, cleaning, and maintaining their living environment. These tasks can provide exercise opportunities that improve cardiovascular health, strength, and flexibility.
3. **Stress Reduction:** Studies have shown that spending time with animals can reduce stress levels and promote a sense of calmness. The soothing presence of chickens and the tranquility of observing them can have a positive impact on mental well-being.
4. **Outdoor Exposure:** Owning chickens encourages spending time outdoors, which provides exposure to sunlight and fresh air. Sunlight exposure helps the body produce vitamin D, which is crucial for bone health and supports the immune system.

Emotional and Mental Well-being:

Caring for chickens can have significant emotional and mental health benefits:

1. **Companionship:** Chickens can provide companionship, especially for individuals who may feel lonely or isolated. The social interaction and bond formed with these intelligent creatures can alleviate feelings of loneliness and boost overall well-being.
2. **Therapeutic Effects:** Many people find solace in the presence of animals. The act of nurturing and connecting with chickens can be therapeutic, reducing anxiety, depression, and other mental health issues.
3. **Teaching Responsibility:** Raising chickens can teach children and adults alike about responsibility, empathy, and compassion. Nurturing living creatures fosters a sense of purpose and fulfillment, enhancing self-esteem and mental resilience.

Potential Risks and Precautions:

While the benefits of chicken ownership are numerous, it is essential to be aware of potential risks and take necessary precautions:

1. **Zoonotic Diseases:** Some diseases can be transmitted between chickens and humans. Examples include salmonella, campylobacter, and avian influenza. Proper hygiene practices, such as regular handwashing, wearing protective clothing, and maintaining a clean coop, can mitigate these risks.
2. **Allergies:** Some individuals may develop allergies to chicken feathers, dander, or dust. If you or a family member have known allergies, consult with a healthcare professional before introducing chickens into your environment.
3. **Occupational Hazards**: Handling chickens and their droppings can expose owners to various occupational hazards, such as respiratory issues from inhaling dust or bacteria. Wearing protective masks, gloves, and appropriate clothing can minimize these risks.
4. **Biosecurity:** Maintaining strict biosecurity measures is crucial to prevent the spread of diseases among your flock and to protect human health. Implementing practices like quarantine, regular vaccinations, and limited visitor access can help maintain a healthy environment for both chickens and owners.

Chapter 18 explored the connection between your chickens and your health. Raising chickens can provide numerous physical, emotional, and mental health benefits, including access to fresh eggs, increased physical activity, stress reduction, companionship, and therapeutic effects. However, it is crucial to be aware of potential risks and take necessary precautions to ensure the well-being of both chickens and humans. By implementing proper hygiene practices, being mindful of allergies, taking precautions against zoonotic diseases, and maintaining biosecurity, you can enjoy the many advantages of owning chickens while safeguarding your health.

Bacterial Infections You Can Get from Chickens

Chickens are one of the most commonly kept livestock animals worldwide, providing meat and eggs to millions of people. While chickens are generally healthy animals, they can harbor certain bacteria that have the potential to cause infections in humans. In this article, we will explore some of the bacterial infections that can be transmitted from chickens to humans and discuss their symptoms, prevention, and treatment options.

1. **Salmonellosis:** Salmonellosis is one of the most well-known bacterial infections associated with chickens. Salmonella bacteria can contaminate eggs, poultry meat, and the environment in which chickens are raised. In humans, salmonellosis can cause diarrhea, abdominal pain, fever, and vomiting. Proper cooking and handling of poultry products, along with good hygiene practices, can significantly reduce the risk of salmonella infection.
2. **Campylobacteriosis:** Campylobacteriosis is another common bacterial infection linked to chickens. Campylobacter bacteria can be present in the intestines of chickens without causing any noticeable symptoms in the birds. However, if humans consume contaminated poultry products, it can lead to gastrointestinal illness characterized by diarrhea, cramping, and fever. Thoroughly cooking poultry, preventing cross-contamination, and practicing good hand hygiene are crucial in preventing Campylobacter infections.

E. **coli Infections:** Certain strains of Escherichia coli (E. coli) bacteria can be found in the intestinal tract of chickens. These bacteria can contaminate poultry products and, if ingested by humans, can cause food poisoning. Symptoms of E. coli infection include severe abdominal cramps, diarrhea (sometimes bloody), and vomiting. Proper cooking and handling of poultry, along with effective handwashing, are essential preventive measures.

3. **Clostridium perfringens**: Clostridium perfringens is a bacteria commonly found in the environment, including the intestines of chickens. Consumption of improperly cooked or stored poultry dishes can lead to clostridium perfringens food poisoning. Symptoms include abdominal pain, diarrhea, and sometimes nausea. Ensuring proper cooking, refrigeration, and reheating practices can help prevent this infection.
4. **Pasteurellosis:** Pasteurellosis is a bacterial infection caused by the Pasteurella multocida bacterium, which is often found in the respiratory tract of chickens. Although primarily affecting poultry, humans can contract the infection through close contact with sick birds or handling contaminated materials. Symptoms may include fever, headache, difficulty breathing, and swollen lymph nodes. Prompt medical attention is necessary if pasteurellosis is suspected.

Prevention and Control Measures:

1. Practice good hygiene, including regular handwashing with soap and water after handling chickens or poultry products.
2. Cook poultry thoroughly, ensuring it reaches an internal temperature of at least 165°F (74°C) to kill bacteria.

3. Prevent cross-contamination by using separate cutting boards, utensils, and plates for raw and cooked poultry.
4. Store poultry at appropriate temperatures to prevent bacterial growth.
5. Avoid contact with sick or dead chickens and wear protective clothing when handling birds.

Treatment Options: If you suspect a bacterial infection from chickens, it is important to seek medical attention promptly. Healthcare professionals may prescribe appropriate antibiotics to treat the infection and relieve symptoms. It is crucial to complete the full course of antibiotics as prescribed to ensure complete eradication of the bacteria from the body.

While chickens are valuable sources of meat and eggs, it is essential to be aware of the potential bacterial infections that can be transmitted from these birds to humans. By following proper hygiene practices, implementing effective prevention measures, and ensuring thorough cooking of poultry products, the risk of contracting bacterial infections can be significantly reduced. It is always advisable to consult a healthcare professional if symptoms of infection arise after exposure to chickens or poultry products.

What You Can Get from Cleaning Chicken Coops

Keeping chickens is a popular hobby and an integral part of many agricultural practices. However, maintaining a clean and healthy chicken coop is crucial to ensuring the well-being of both the chickens and those who care for them. Cleaning chicken coops regularly helps to prevent the buildup of waste, bacteria, and other potential health hazards. In this wide content, we will focus on two specific risks associated with cleaning chicken coops: histoplasmosis and farmer's lung.

Histoplasmosis is a fungal infection caused by the inhalation of spores from the fungus Histoplasma capsulatum, which is commonly found in soil contaminated by bird or bat droppings. When chicken owners clean their coops, they may unknowingly disturb dried droppings that contain these fungal spores. Once disturbed, the spores can become airborne and easily inhaled.

The symptoms of histoplasmosis can vary, ranging from mild flu-like symptoms to severe respiratory problems. Common signs include fever, cough, chest pain, fatigue, and joint pain. In most cases, healthy individuals with mild infections recover without specific treatment. However, individuals with weakened immune systems or chronic lung conditions may develop more severe forms of the disease, requiring medical intervention. To minimize the risk of contracting histoplasmosis when cleaning chicken coops, it is crucial to take appropriate precautions, such as wearing respiratory protection, using gloves, and ensuring proper ventilation.

Farmer's lung, also known as hypersensitivity pneumonitis, is another respiratory condition that can be linked to cleaning chicken coops. It is an allergic reaction to the inhalation of various organic particles, including mold spores, bacteria, fungi, and dust found in the coop environment. When chicken owners disturb bedding materials, dried feces, feathers, and other organic matter during cleaning, these particles become airborne, leading to potential exposure.

The symptoms of farmer's lung typically include cough, shortness of breath, chest tightness, fatigue, and fever. These symptoms may develop hours after exposure and can worsen over time if the individual continues to be exposed to the allergens. Long-term exposure to the causative agents can cause irreversible lung damage. Prevention of farmer's lung involves using protective equipment, such as respiratory masks, goggles, and gloves, as well as ensuring proper ventilation during coop cleaning.

To maintain a healthy environment while cleaning chicken coops, here are some additional tips:

1. **Schedule regular cleanings:** Establish a cleaning routine to prevent the accumulation of waste materials in the coop. Remove soiled bedding, droppings, and uneaten food regularly to minimize the potential for respiratory irritants and pathogens.
2. **Use appropriate cleaning agents:** Choose disinfectants and cleaning solutions specifically designed for use in poultry environments. Avoid using harsh chemicals that can be harmful to both humans and chickens.
3. **Minimize dust and airborne particles:** Wet down bedding materials before removing them to reduce the dispersion of allergens and irritants into the air. Consider using a dust mask or respirator to protect yourself from inhaling particles.
4. **Maintain proper ventilation:** Ensure that the coop has adequate airflow and ventilation systems in place to prevent the buildup of stale air and excessive moisture. Good ventilation helps to reduce the concentration of airborne contaminants.
5. **Practice good hygiene:** Wash your hands thoroughly after handling chickens, cleaning coops, or coming into contact with any potentially contaminated materials. This simple practice helps to minimize the risk of spreading pathogens or other harmful substances.

Remember, the health and safety of both chickens and chicken owners are interconnected. By understanding and addressing the risks associated with cleaning chicken coops, you can create a safer environment for everyone involved. Stay informed, take necessary precautions, and enjoy the rewards of raising healthy and happy chickens.

How to Protect Yourself

Keeping chickens can be a rewarding and enjoyable experience, but it also comes with the responsibility of safeguarding their health. Just like any other animal, chickens are susceptible to various diseases and illnesses. However, with proper knowledge and proactive measures, you can protect your feathered friends and ensure their well-being. In this guide, we will explore essential practices and strategies to help you protect yourself and your flock from potential health risks.

Biosecurity Measures:

Biosecurity Measures is crucial in preventing the spread of diseases among chickens. Implement the following practices to maintain a healthy environment:

1. **Restricted Access:** Limit access to your chicken coop and run to authorized individuals

only. This reduces the risk of introducing diseases through contaminated equipment or footwear.
2. **Quarantine:** When introducing new chickens to your flock, isolate them in a separate area for a minimum of 30 days. This helps identify any potential health issues before integrating them with the existing flock.
3. **Cleanliness and Hygiene:** Regularly clean and disinfect your coop and equipment. Remove droppings, replace bedding, and ensure fresh water and feed are available. Keep wild birds, rodents, and pests away from the coop, as they can carry diseases.
4. **Footwear and Clothing:** Use dedicated footwear and clothing when tending to your chickens. This prevents cross-contamination from other areas.

Vaccinations:

Consult a veterinarian or poultry expert to determine the appropriate vaccinations for your flock. Vaccines can provide immunity against common poultry diseases such as Newcastle disease, infectious bronchitis, and Marek's disease. Follow the recommended vaccination schedule to ensure optimal protection.

Nutritional Health:

Maintaining a balanced and nutritious diet is essential for strong immunity and overall health. Provide your chickens with high-quality feed that meets their specific nutritional requirements. Supplement their diet with fresh fruits, vegetables, and grit to promote optimal digestion.

Parasite Control:

Internal and external parasites can pose significant threats to chicken health. Regularly inspect your flock for signs of parasites such as mites, lice, worms, or ticks. Administer appropriate treatments and follow recommended protocols for parasite control.

Environmental Considerations:

Create a clean and comfortable environment for your chickens:
1. **Ventilation:** Ensure proper airflow in the coop to prevent respiratory issues. Good ventilation helps remove moisture and ammonia, promoting a healthy environment.
2. **Temperature Regulation:** Maintain suitable temperatures according to the breed and weather conditions. Provide shade in hot weather and implement heating measures during colder seasons.
3. **Space and Roosting:** Allow ample space for each chicken to minimize stress and prevent overcrowding. Provide suitable roosting options to encourage natural behavior and minimize foot and leg problems.

Early Detection and Treatment:

Regularly observe your flock for any signs of illness, such as changes in behavior, appetite, or appearance. Consult a veterinarian if you notice any unusual symptoms. Early detection and prompt treatment can prevent the spread of diseases and increase the chances of recovery.

Education and Networking:

Stay updated on the latest advancements in chicken health by attending workshops, seminars, or online forums. Networking with fellow chicken keepers and professionals allows you to share experiences and gain valuable insights into disease prevention and management.

Protecting your chickens' health is crucial for their well-being and productivity. By implementing biosecurity measures, vaccinations, proper nutrition, parasite control, and maintaining a suitable environment, you can significantly reduce the risk of diseases and ensure a healthy flock. Regular monitoring, early detection, and prompt treatment are essential practices to safeguard your chickens. Remember, knowledge and proactive measures are key to protecting yourself and your feathered companions.

Conclusion

In conclusion, the "Chicken Health Bible" serves as an invaluable resource for poultry enthusiasts, farmers, and anyone interested in raising healthy chickens. Throughout this comprehensive guide, we have explored various aspects of chicken health, ranging from preventative measures to identifying and treating common ailments. By following the guidelines outlined in the book, individuals can ensure the well-being of their flock, promote optimal growth and productivity, and ultimately enjoy the rewards of successful chicken rearing.

One of the key takeaways from the "Chicken Health Bible" is the importance of proactive care and preventive measures. By implementing a robust biosecurity plan, maintaining a clean and sanitary environment, and providing a balanced diet, chicken owners can significantly reduce the risk of disease outbreaks. Regular vaccinations, deworming, and health checks are essential components of a preventative approach, ensuring that the flock remains in good health and minimizing the need for intensive treatments in the future.

Furthermore, the "Chicken Health Bible" emphasizes the significance of early detection and prompt action when it comes to addressing health issues. By being vigilant and closely monitoring the behavior, appearance, and egg production of the chickens, owners can identify potential problems at their earliest stages. The book provides detailed information on recognizing common ailments, such as respiratory infections, parasitic infestations, or nutritional deficiencies, and offers comprehensive guidance on appropriate treatment options.

Additionally, the "Chicken Health Bible" emphasizes the importance of seeking professional advice and consulting a veterinarian when faced with complex or severe health issues. While the book provides a wealth of information, it is crucial to remember that each chicken is unique, and some cases may require specific expertise. Veterinary guidance ensures accurate diagnoses, tailored treatment plans, and the best possible outcomes for the birds.

The "Chicken Health Bible" also promotes the well-being of chickens by encouraging ethical and humane practices. It highlights the significance of providing appropriate housing, sufficient space, and enrichments that stimulate natural behaviors. Additionally, the book emphasizes the importance of responsible antibiotic use, advocating for alternative methods and natural remedies whenever possible to minimize the risk of antibiotic resistance.

In conclusion, the "Chicken Health Bible" is a comprehensive and practical guide that equips individuals with the knowledge and tools necessary to maintain the health and well-being of their chickens. By following the principles outlined in this book, chicken owners can ensure a thriving flock, enjoy the benefits of sustainable poultry farming, and promote the overall welfare of these fascinating and valuable creatures. With its wealth of information, practical tips, and emphasis on preventive care, the "Chicken Health Bible" is an essential resource for anyone invested in the health and happiness of their chickens.

Made in the USA
Monee, IL
08 September 2023